THE BRAIN HEALTH
COOKBOOK

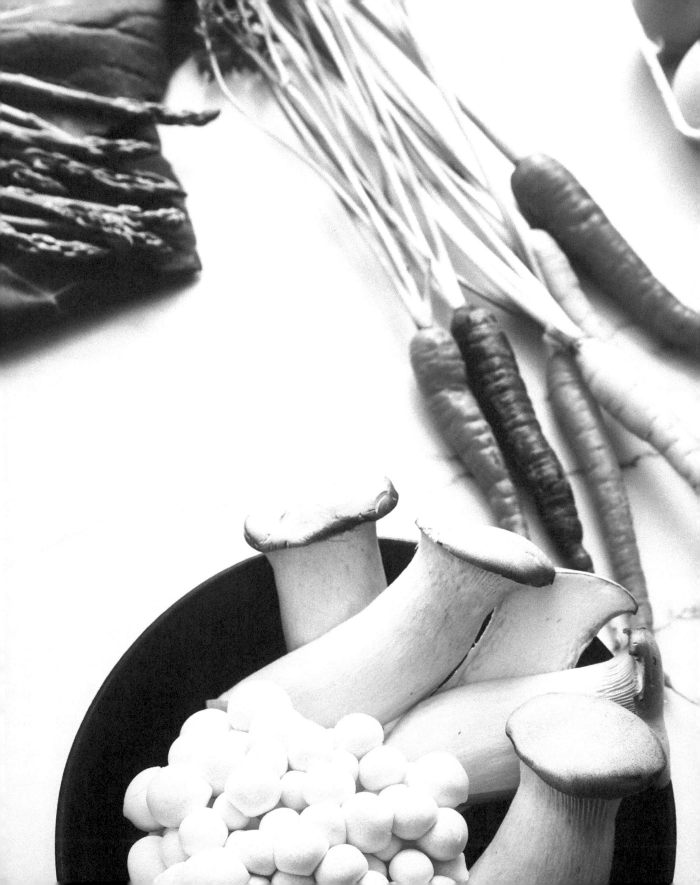

THE
BRAIN HEALTH
COOKBOOK

MIND Diet Recipes to Prevent Disease and Enhance Cognitive Power

Julie Andrews, MS, RDN, CD
Photography by Alicia Cho

ROCKRIDGE PRESS

To each and every one of you who picks up this book
and crafts something delicious from it.
I hope you enjoy every morsel.

Interior and Cover Designer: Mando Daniel
Art Producer: Karen Williams
Editor: Rachelle Cihonski
Production Editor: Ruth Sakata Corley

Photography ©2020 Alicia Cho. Food styling by Ashley Nevarez. Prop styling: Alicia Cho and Ashley Nevarez. Author photo courtesy of ©Julie Andrews.

ISBN: Print 978-1-64611-517-4 | eBook 978-1-64611-518-1

R0

CONTENTS

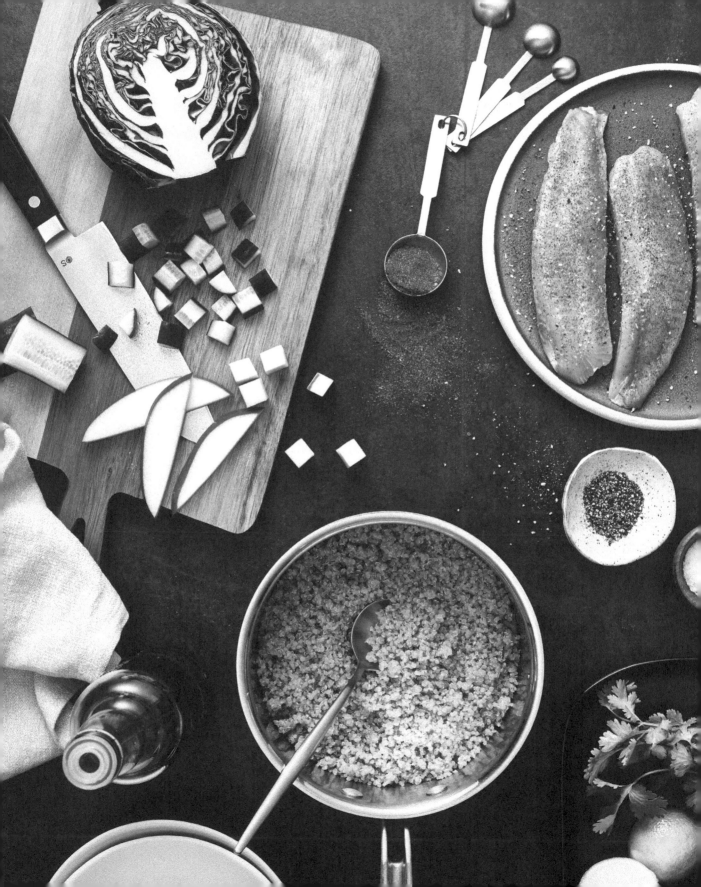

INTRODUCTION

Finding balance is truly one of the most important things we can do for our physical and mental well-being, but it's also one of the most difficult to master. As a chef and registered dietitian, I have spent many years working with people who want to maintain or achieve good health but want to do it in a way that is satisfying, enjoyable, and practical.

One of the most rewarding experiences of my career has been teaching people how to prevent and manage chronic conditions through healthy cooking, and that's because I've seen the positive impact it has on their lives. These experiences have shaped my philosophy and perspective surrounding what healthy cooking and eating really means, which may be different from what you'd expect. I believe that cooking (mostly) from scratch in simple ways, using (mostly) wholesome and nourishing ingredients is the key to building a balanced diet and having a positive relationship with food.

We often associate scratch cooking with spending hours in the kitchen on time-intensive recipes that require expert culinary skills, but in reality, my style of scratch cooking is using everyday ingredients and simple cooking techniques that everyone can master and that result in flavorful meals the entire family will love. I also believe that having a balanced eating style and making good food choices doesn't have to be an all-or-nothing approach, and that we can enjoy all foods without sabotaging our health goals. (Yes, even a donut won't hurt every once in a while.) Sure, we'll focus on incorporating nourishing foods like vegetables, fruits, beans, salmon, and olive oil into your diet on a regular basis because we know our health will benefit, but I'll also show you how to enjoy some of your other favorite foods as part of a healthy diet. After all, my intention is to help you create a balanced lifestyle that you can maintain for the rest of your life.

With that said, each and every recipe in this cookbook is based around this philosophy and developed using the latest evidenced-based recommendations for preserving brain health and preventing cognitive decline. I've translated the science behind the MIND diet into easy and scrumptious recipes and cooking tips that can help you achieve a healthy, balanced, and nourishing eating style with truly delicious foods. The recipes and guidelines in this book also consider the nutrition and lifestyle recommendations for reducing the risk of and managing conditions such as obesity, type 2 diabetes, and cardiovascular disease, because of their connection to cognitive decline and neurodegenerative diseases.

Paired with the science behind other important aspects of holistic well-being, such as stress management, adequate sleep and hydration, positive social interactions, intellectual pursuits, and regular physical activity, this book is the ultimate guide to preserving cognition and achieving good overall health in a realistic way. So, let's get started!

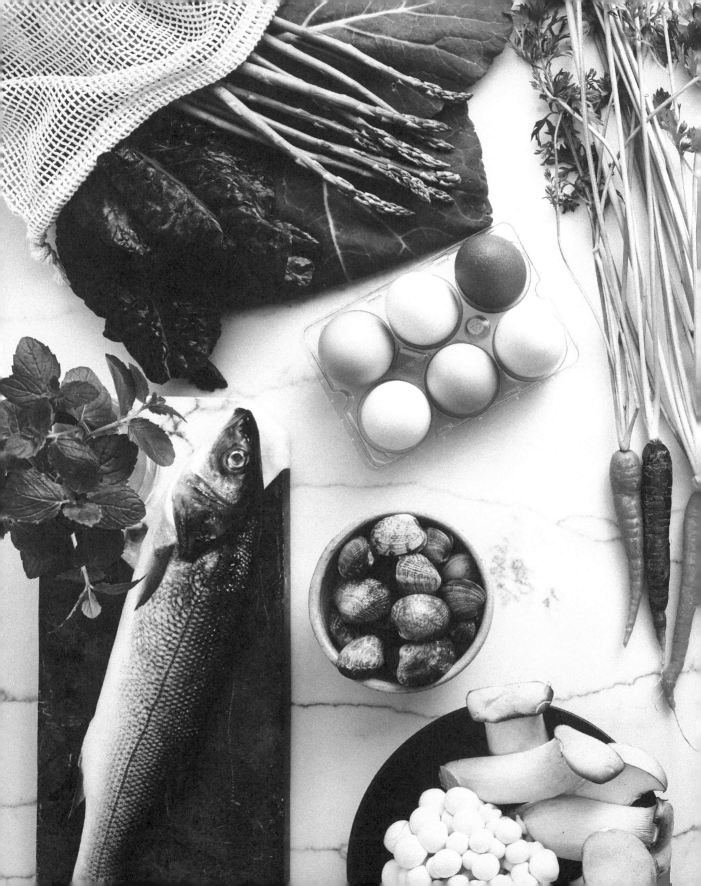

ALL ABOUT BRAIN HEALTH

PART ONE

The brain is one of the most complex organs in the human body. It is constantly at work, even while you're asleep—controlling your ability to think, talk, read, feel, see, hear, move, learn, remember, and breathe. The brain communicates with systems throughout the body via neurons, or nerve cells, so it's no surprise that your brain function impacts your entire body.

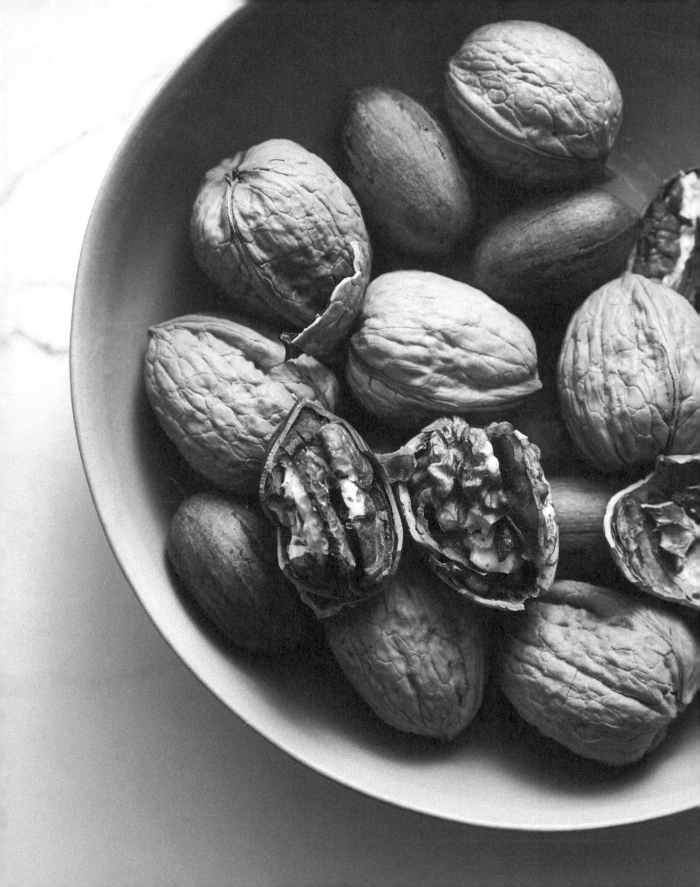

CHAPTER ONE
Inside Your Head

In our crazy, busy world, it's no wonder many of us have trouble focusing, staying energized, and maintaining a consistent mood. Most of us are searching for ways to preserve brain efficiency and energy levels, and to regulate our mood, especially as we age, and we still have much to learn regarding the connection between food and brain health. Researchers have become increasingly interested in the way our lifestyle impacts our ability to stay mentally sharp, and how that impacts our risk of developing neurodegenerative conditions, which are those that cause the loss of structure and function of neurons.

Depending on factors such as age, genetics, lifestyle, and diet, your brain can suffer a buildup of harmful inflammatory substances that can damage brain tissue and neurons, diminishing its ability to carry out normal functions. Those functions could be everything from remembering to pick up the kids at school to taking your contact lenses out at night, or from holding a thoughtful conversation to giving a presentation at work.

Inflammation, at its core, is our body's reaction when it is invaded by a substance or object our body identifies as harmful. Acute inflammation occurs, for example, when you scrape your knee and the area becomes red and swollen. Your body sends immune cells to heal the wound and stop you from getting an infection. Chronic inflammation, however, is a different story. It occurs at a low level over a long period of time, and when it goes unchecked, the immune system responds by attacking nearby organs and tissues. Chronic inflammation can be caused by a poor diet, tobacco use, excessive alcohol consumption, and chronic stress, to name a few. Research has linked chronic inflammation to diseases such as cancer, heart disease, type 2 diabetes, obesity, and neurodegenerative diseases like Alzheimer's disease.

For many years, surprisingly, health experts didn't connect nutrition with brain health, but the good news is that researchers now know how important it is to fuel your body with nutritious foods and practice other healthy habits in order to support your brain as you age. The healthy habits we'll discuss throughout this book can help reduce your risk of developing dementia and neurological diseases like Alzheimer's disease, and I'll also show you how nutrition and lifestyle can support cognitive function, brain efficiency, energy levels, and mood.

YOUR BRAIN HEALTH

As you age, it's common to notice some changes related to communication, memory, and overall cognition. That's because the brain goes through physical changes, such as a loss of tissue volume (shrinkage), a loss of nerve cells, and a buildup of waste products; often as the result of chronic inflammation. According to the Harvard Medical School, however, not all changes in your brain over time are negative. You may notice some improvements in cognition, such as a greater ability to sort through thoughts, ideas, and concepts from a holistic viewpoint, and to understand complex issues and how they impact the world. As they say: with age comes wisdom. This may be because dendrites, the tree-like ends of neurons that receive communication, sprout and lengthen, which strengthens connections between separate parts of the brain. Several factors, like genetics, diet, and lifestyle, impact how your brain changes and how those changes affect you on a day-to-day basis.

Your Age and Genetics

There are many things you can do to help improve and protect your brain health, but there are two factors you simply cannot control: genetics and the fact that you have a birthday each year. Starting in mid-life, several things begin to happen. The volume of your brain decreases, communication between neurons may ebb, and blood flow to the brain may decrease.

According to the National Institutes of Health (NIH), brain volume decreases at a rate of around 5 percent per decade after age 40, with the rate of decline possibly increasing once you get to age 70. As the area that surrounds and protects the nerve fibers, called the myelin sheath, wears down, the communication speed between neurons slows. As nerve cells break down, waste products can build up in the brain tissue. The shrinkage of blood vessels causes the rate of blood flow to decrease, which can often lead to a rise in blood pressure and increased risk of stroke.

Researchers at the Mayo Clinic have also identified several genes associated with Alzheimer's disease. Some of them are considered risk genes, which increase your likelihood of developing the disease, and others, while rare, are called deterministic genes that guarantee development of the disease at some point in life. The most common type of Alzheimer's disease, called late-onset Alzheimer's, occurs after the age of 65 and is associated with a gene called apolipoprotein E (APOE). Having this gene affects risk, but research shows that not everyone who has the gene develops Alzheimer's disease, suggesting this specific gene is not itself a cause.

However, researchers believe a specific APOE allele, noted as APOE e4, increases the carrier's risk of developing late-onset Alzheimer's disease. There are many other genes that may impact your risk of developing Alzheimer's disease, but more research is needed. Because the research on genes related to Alzheimer's disease is relatively new, experts don't currently suggest genetic testing for most people.

It's easy to feel a loss of control over how your brain ages, especially if you have a family history of Alzheimer's disease or dementia. But the good news is you can control your diet and lifestyle, which can have a big—and positive—impact on your brain health.

Contributing Conditions

Inflammation is a primary concern for many, if not all, chronic conditions. A growing body of research suggests that the same risk factors for diseases such as type 2 diabetes, prediabetes, heart disease, hypertension, and obesity—collectively known as metabolic syndrome—are also the same for neurological diseases like Alzheimer's disease.

Evidence shows a strong relationship between the brain and the cardiovascular system. The heart feeds oxygen to all parts of the body, including the brain, therefore cardiovascular health heavily impacts brain health. Some of the same lifestyle strategies that protect the heart may also protect the brain; strategies such as not smoking, moderate to low alcohol intake, maintaining a nutritious diet with key nutrients, participating in regular physical activity, and maintaining a healthy weight, blood glucose levels, and blood cholesterol levels. Studies show that heart disease, type 2 diabetes, obesity, depression, and lack of participation in socially and mentally stimulating activities may also increase your risk of Alzheimer's disease, dementia, and cognitive decline.

The connection between metabolic syndrome and brain health (as well as other chronic conditions) is strong, so it's important to take a holistic approach to the prevention and treatment of these conditions.

ALZHEIMER'S, DEMENTIA, AND MENTAL DECLINE

Alzheimer's disease, dementia, and mental decline manifest in similar ways and can be difficult to differentiate from one another. Alzheimer's is a neurological disease that affects memory and cognition, whereas dementia is a group of symptoms related to memory, communication, problem-solving, and thinking skills. Mental decline, also known as cognitive decline, is an impairment in brain function that may resolve or progress over time. We will address each of these conditions in more depth, then address how diet and lifestyle can affect all three.

Alzheimer's Disease

The most common myth of Alzheimer's disease is that it's a condition of old age. Age is certainly a risk factor, but the symptoms of Alzheimer's are not characteristic of aging. It's a type of dementia that progresses over time, causing a disruption in memory, thinking, and behavior due to a loss of communication between nerve cells. The National Institute on Aging describes it as the formation of abnormal clumps, called amyloid plaques; and bundles of fibers, called neurofibrillary tangles, that break the connection between nerve cells and/or cause them to die. The damage appears to first take place in the hippocampus, which is the part of the brain responsible for memories, and then progresses to other parts of the brain. What's to blame for all this trouble? Researchers believe oxidation from chronic inflammation and buildup of harmful free radicals in the brain kick-starts the plaque and tangle formations.

Signs of slight memory loss, like forgetting a regularly scheduled appointment, may be a first sign of the early stages of disease. As the disease progresses, the ability to stay focused, hold a conversation, or recall a recent event may begin to diminish. We've all heard stories about people with Alzheimer's disease who wander off, become confused and disoriented, only to be found close by but unable to find their way home. Alzheimer's can create some very disorienting moments, which are commonly followed by changes in mood and behavior, and then the loss of mobility, making everyday tasks like eating and walking difficult.

Some researchers have proposed labeling Alzheimer's disease as "type 3 diabetes" because evidence suggests Alzheimer's disease may be triggered by a type of insulin resistance, insulin-like growth factor dysfunction, and impaired insulin signaling, specifically in the brain, causing a decrease in the brain's ability to metabolize sugar efficiently. Researchers believe the gene APOE e4 may influence this process. It's important to note that someone with type 1 or type 2 diabetes likely has a higher risk of developing brain-specific insulin resistance and insulin deficiency, among other risk factors. It may also be possible that insulin therapy could halt the progression of cognitive impairment. In fact, a 2016 National Institutes of Health pilot study showed intranasal insulin used in the treatment of mild cognitive impairment and early stage Alzheimer's disease showed significant improvements in learning, memory, and cognition. However, more research is needed.

Dementia

Dementia is not a disease, but a group of symptoms such as loss of memory, changes in communication and language, loss of focus and attention, changes in reasoning and judgement, and visual changes. Some may experience a change in personality and become more aggressive and irritable. They may forget names, lose their car keys, have trouble paying bills and making meals, forget their way home, and get frustrated easily over small tasks. Most cases of dementia are progressive, starting with mild symptoms that worsen over time. While everyone loses neurons as they age, those with dementia experience far greater loss. At the end stages, those with dementia often depend on a full-time caretaker in order to carry out activities of daily living.

Alzheimer's disease is the most common cause of dementia, but vascular dementia, Lewy body dementia, and frontotemporal disorders can also be culprits. According to the NIH, most people with dementia have mixed dementia, which is a combination of two or more types.

A patient's medical history, a physical examination, a review of symptoms, and lab tests are required to make a diagnosis of Alzheimer's or dementia. There is no cure for dementia, but as with Alzheimer's, there are treatments and medications available that may help improve quality of life and manage symptoms. There are also some key lifestyle choices that you can make, including what you eat, that can work to reduce your risk of developing dementia.

Mental Decline

Mental decline, also known as cognitive impairment or cognitive decline, may include problems with diminishing memory, learning abilities, concentration, and decision-making skills, as well as changes in mood. Someone with cognitive decline may easily forget to go to a doctor's appointment, have trouble recalling a family gathering, or misplace common items like their glasses, but the changes are not significant enough to interfere with normal life. Those with cognitive decline may also experience depression, anxiety, apathy, and irritability. Symptoms of cognitive decline may worsen over time and indicate increased risk of developing Alzheimer's disease or dementia, but studies show that not everyone with cognitive decline develops Alzheimer's disease or dementia. Everyone loses some of their cognitive function naturally as they age, but symptoms beyond a temporary lapse of memory are a reason for concern. If you or a family member feels their symptoms are worsening or do not improve, it's wise to seek help from your doctor.

THE GUT-BRAIN CONNECTION

Emerging research links dysbiosis of the gut microbiota (an imbalance of the bacteria living in your gut) and inflammatory diseases of the neurological system, such as Alzheimer's disease. A 2019 study in the *Journal of Neurogastroenterology and Motility* explained that the gut-brain axis allows communication back and forth between the central nervous system (CNS) and the gastrointestinal system. When it becomes disturbed and unbalanced, it can cause chronic inflammation and contribute to the pathogenesis of Alzheimer's disease. Common causes of dysbiosis include excessive alcohol intake, antibiotic use, high levels of stress or anxiety, and a poor diet. More research is needed, but experts recommend supporting a healthy gut microbiota by consuming nutritious foods like vegetables and fish, and fermented foods like yogurt, kefir, miso, sourdough bread, sauerkraut, kimchi, tempeh, and kombucha. Probiotic and prebiotic supplements may also be helpful.

HOW DIET AFFECTS YOUR BRAIN

Most of us are aware that nutrition can impact our health in certain ways, for example, eating adequate fiber can improve digestion, or counting calories can help with weight loss, but it wasn't until several years ago that we really started to connect diet with brain health. We now know that a few specific nutrients can preserve cognition, while other nutrients can hinder it. The former include omega-3 fatty acids, vitamin E, B vitamins, flavonoids, lutein, and beta carotene. Newer research suggests that vitamins C and D and choline may also be supportive of brain function. A lack of these nutrients in our diet, plus eating too much refined sugar and saturated and trans fats has been linked to chronic inflammation and neurodegenerative diseases like Alzheimer's. The brain requires a constant source of high-quality fuel in order to support its functions, and we'll dig deeper into the food recommendations in the next chapter.

Omega-3 Fatty Acids

Omega-3 fatty acids are a hallmark of a brain- and heart-healthy diet, and for good reason. A large body of evidence shows that the benefits of adequate omega-3 consumption include less inflammation in the body, reduced risk of cardiovascular disease and blood clots, lower triglycerides and blood pressure, prevention of plaque formation in the arteries, healthy arterial structure and increased levels of high-density lipoprotein (HDL), i.e., "good" cholesterol levels.

The three main types of omega-3 fatty acids include alpha linoleic acid (ALA), eicosapentaenoic acid (EPA), and docosahexaenoic acid (DHA). Canola, flaxseed, and soybean oils; flax and chia seeds; and walnuts are all good sources of ALA, which is found in plant foods. Fatty fish such as mackerel, salmon, trout, and tuna are the best sources of DHA and EPA. The body cannot manufacture ALA on its own, making it an essential nutrient that must be consumed in the diet. It is possible for the body to convert ALA to DHA and EPA, but only in small amounts, which is why it's good to dine on both plant- and fish-based sources of omega-3s, with an emphasis on the fish.

DHA is the most abundant fat in the brain and is used to carry out its functions, making DHA the crown jewel of the omega-3s when it comes to brain health. As we age, years of oxidative stress can also cause DHA levels to decrease. A review in the journal *Nutrients*, as well as many other studies, have shown that DHA's role in membrane and neurotransmitter conduction in the brain makes it protective against the development of Alzheimer's disease. Low omega-3 intake may also predispose certain people to depression and anxiety, according to a 2018 study in *Frontiers in Physiology*.

Vitamin E

Vitamin E, primarily in the form of alpha-tocopherol, is found in nuts, seeds, green vegetables, some fortified grains, and vegetable oils. We've likely all heard vitamin E is great for both the immune and cardiovascular systems, but it's also been linked to improved brain health. But what makes it so special? Well, its main job is to protect the brain from a build-up of free radicals that can damage healthy brain cells and cause inflammation. It also fights off invading bacteria and viruses. In addition, it helps the blood clot and prevents plaque build-up in the arteries. Basically, you can think of it as a scavenger of substances that can harm your brain, heart, and immune system, which all work together.

While studies on high-dose supplementation of vitamin E are inconclusive, researchers believe a diet rich in vitamin E, among other key nutrients, can have a positive impact on overall brain health. A 2017 study in the journal *Alzheimer's and Dementia* showed that levels of alpha-tocopherol were significantly lower in people who were diagnosed with Alzheimer's disease, and a 2014 study in *Food and Public Health* suggested that oxidative damage and inflammation of the brain tissue can contribute to mental disorders such as anxiety, depression, mild cognitive impairment, and attention-deficit/hyperactivity disorder (ADHD), to name a few.

VITAMIN C'S ROLE

Vitamin C is well-known for carrying out antioxidant functions in the body. In the brain, it heavily accumulates in neurons, synthesizes neurotransmitters, and protects the myelin sheath, making it a crucial nutrient for cognitive performance. Studies show that a deficiency of vitamin C can cause oxidative damage in the brain, and we also know that vitamin C supports the functions of vitamin E. Food sources of vitamin C include mango, pineapple, melons, citrus fruit, berries, kiwi, Brussels sprouts, cauliflower, broccoli, bell peppers, spinach and other leafy greens, sweet and white potatoes, winter squash, and tomatoes.

B Vitamins

The eight water-soluble B vitamins are considered a complex because they work together to carry out basic metabolic tasks. Each has a unique role that impacts your energy level, metabolism, immune system, and cell health. The B vitamins folate, B_6, and B_{12} are of particular interest because they are necessary in the development and maintenance of brain function. A 2015 review in *Proceedings of the Nutrition Society* concluded that these three B vitamins are essential for brain health across all age groups. According to the Cleveland Clinic, B vitamins may help prevent dementia because they boost the production of neurotransmitters that deliver messages between neurons in the brain and the rest of the body, and without adequate supply, we are at a greater risk of memory loss, cognitive decline, and neurodegenerative diseases. You can find folate in whole grains, beans, fruits, vegetables, and fortified breakfast cereals and grain products. Vitamin B_6 is found in poultry, fish, beans, oranges, cantaloupe, dark leafy green vegetables, and fortified breakfast cereals. Animal products like fish, poultry, red meat, eggs, dairy—and some fortified breakfast cereals—are great sources of vitamin B_{12}.

Flavonoids

In a 2019 study in *Frontiers in Aging Neuroscience*, it was concluded that consumption of flavonoid-rich foods can lessen age-related decline in cognition, promote new cell growth in the hippocampus, restore memory functions, and slow the development of conditions associated with dementia. The study also concluded that flavonoids inhibit neuronal cell death induced by free radicals and beta amyloid proteins, a hallmark of Alzheimer's disease. Flavonoids may also play a role in helping the vascular system work properly. There are many subclasses of naturally anti-inflammatory and antioxidant-rich flavonoids, and some sources include berries, teas, red wine, cocoa, legumes, soybeans, and some fruits, vegetables, and herbs.

Lutein

Lutein is a carotenoid with antioxidant and anti-inflammatory properties found in egg yolks, green leafy vegetables, and other green and yellow vegetables. It is a crucial nutrient for brain development in infants and children and, according to a 2019 review in *Current Developments in Nutrition*, lutein is also a key nutrient for cognitive function in younger and older adults.

Beta Carotene

Beta carotene, a precursor of vitamin A, is a carotenoid found in red, orange, and yellow fruits and vegetables that, when consumed regularly, may help reduce your risk of cognitive decline. A 2019 study in the *European Journal of Nutrition* associated low plasma beta carotene levels in older adults with the diagnosis of Alzheimer's disease.

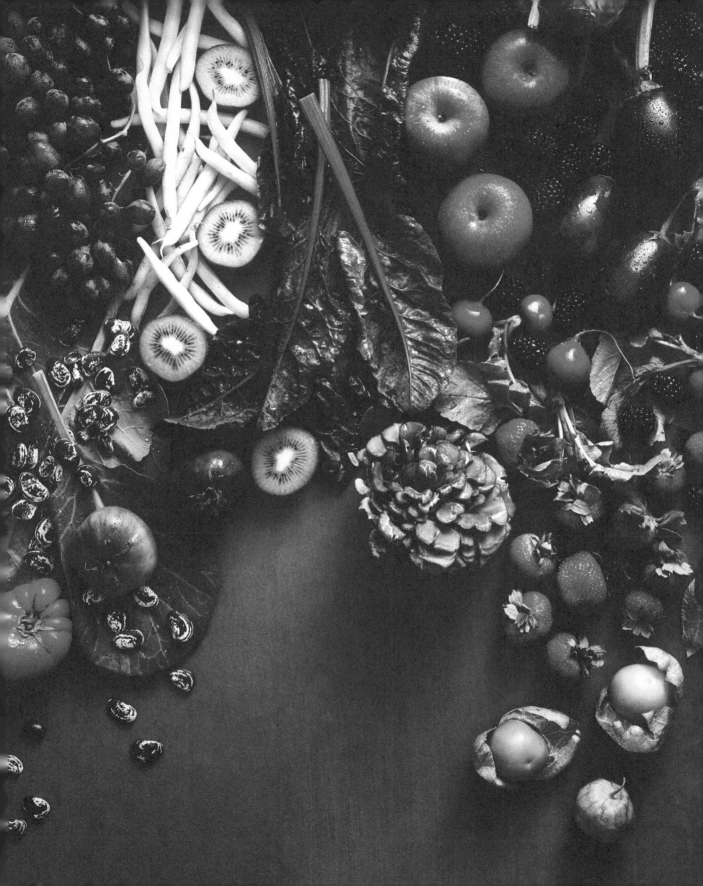

CHAPTER TWO

The MIND Diet

Now that we've discussed the research surrounding key nutrients and their link to brain health, we'll dive deeper into the foods and food groups that contain these brain-healthy nutrients and how often we should eat them to help preserve cognition. This eating pattern, known as the MIND diet, is shown to have a significant impact on brain health and can reduce your risk of developing neurodegenerative diseases. And aside from its powerful impact on brain health, I love this way of eating because it's all-inclusive, easy-to-follow, and loaded with flavorful ingredients. As we go through the next few chapters, you'll see exactly what I mean.

A BRIEF OVERVIEW OF THE DIET

The MIND diet, which stands for Mediterranean-DASH Intervention for Neurodegenerative Delay, is a set of diet and lifestyle recommendations based on promising brain-health research. It combines aspects of the Mediterranean and DASH (Dietary Approaches to Stop Hypertension) diets that best support brain health and reduce the risk of developing Alzheimer's disease and dementia. The Mediterranean diet is based on foods commonly eaten in the countries lining the Mediterranean Sea and is well-known for its heart-health benefits. The DASH diet is a well-balanced, all-inclusive eating plan to help reduce blood pressure and promote heart health. Because of the strong link between heart health and brain health, researchers became interested in how these diets may impact the brain. A 2013 study in the *American Journal of Clinical Nutrition* that covered an 11-year period showed that high adherence to both the Mediterranean and DASH diets was associated with greater levels of cognitive function in elderly women and men. While this study shows the Mediterranean and DASH diets are beneficial to brain health, the MIND diet has an even greater impact on brain health.

The MIND diet takes the recommendations for consumption of brain-healthy nutrients—omega-3 fatty acids, vitamin E, B vitamins, flavonoids, lutein, and beta carotene—and translates them into recommended servings of foods and food groups that are good or great sources of these nutrients. That means you'll eat plenty of leafy green vegetables, low-starch vegetables, berries, whole grains and starchy vegetables, beans and legumes, nuts and seeds, seafood, poultry, and heart-healthy oils. Some of these foods are considered daily foods, meaning you'll eat at least one serving of them every day, and others are considered weekly foods, meaning you'll eat them at least once a week. My main goal is to help you incorporate these foods into your diet, consistent with the MIND diet recommendations, without having to think too hard (pun intended) about getting delicious food on the table.

There are also a handful of foods that, if consumed in excess, can increase your risk of developing neurodegenerative diseases and may contribute to brain inefficiency, low energy levels, and poor mood. These foods include processed meats, red meat, whole-fat dairy, sweets, and fried foods. We will consider these "sometimes foods" because they contain trans fats, saturated fats, and/or refined sugars. In the next sections, I will outline the recommended daily and weekly intake of MIND-friendly foods and, because we live in the real world, how to enjoy the "sometimes foods" in a healthy way.

Mediterranean Diet

The Mediterranean diet focuses on eating a largely plant-based diet, including vegetables, fruits, whole grains, nuts and seeds, beans and legumes, and olive oil. In addition, flavoring dishes with herbs and spices instead of excess salt, enjoying fish and poultry at least twice a week, and drinking red wine in moderation are all common components of the Mediterranean diet.

Extra-virgin olive oil is the primary cooking fat used in the Mediterranean diet. Olive oil contains monounsaturated fats (MUFAs), which are shown to help increase HDL (good) cholesterol levels, and reduce LDL (bad) cholesterol levels in the blood. Fatty fish rich in omega-3 is consumed at least twice a week, with some resources suggesting as many as six servings a week while following the Mediterranean diet. According to the Mayo Clinic, some studies have shown that moderate consumption of red wine can reduce risk of heart disease. But perhaps what makes the Mediterranean diet most unique is that it's not just a diet. A major part of the Mediterranean way of life includes enjoying meals with friends and family, practicing mindful eating habits, and exercising regularly.

There is growing evidence that the risk of developing chronic conditions can be reduced by following the Mediterranean way of eating. According to a 2017 review in *Nutrition Today*, following the Mediterranean diet can reduce risk of Alzheimer's disease, metabolic syndrome, obesity, type 2 diabetes, cardiovascular diseases, and breast and other types of cancers. This isn't surprising, as the Mediterranean diet is loaded with foods rich in omega-3 fatty acids, monounsaturated fats, fiber, vitamins, minerals, and antioxidants; is low in trans and saturated fats and refined carbohydrates; and puts a strong emphasis on a holistic approach to health and well-being.

DASH Diet

The DASH (Dietary Approaches to Stop Hypertension) diet is an all-inclusive eating plan that is centered around consuming a nutritious, well-balanced diet. It forgoes restricting foods and food groups, and instead places its focus on consuming vegetables, fruits, legumes, nuts, seeds, low-fat dairy, whole grains, lean meats, poultry and seafood, and heart-healthy oils. Restrictions include avoiding trans fats and limiting saturated fat and sodium.

The DASH diet is easy to follow and has been shown effective in lowering blood pressure and supporting heart health, resulting in the diet being consistently ranked as a top diet in *U.S. News and World Report*. A study in *Frontiers in Nutrition* concluded that increased blood pressure leads to an increased risk of neurodegeneration, stroke, and gray matter volume loss in the brain, which can lead to cognitive dysfunction. According to a 2014 study in *Neurology* and a 2013 study in *The American Journal of Clinical Nutrition,* higher levels of cognitive function and slower rates of cognitive decline were shown in people adhering to the DASH and Mediterranean diets.

The Best of Both Diets

While following the Mediterranean and DASH diets has been shown to benefit brain health, the MIND diet research shows that following the specific guidelines of the MIND diet has an even greater impact on preserving cognitive health. A 2015 study in the journal *Alzheimer's & Dementia* estimated a 35 percent reduction in Alzheimer's disease risk with moderate adherence to the MIND diet and a 53 percent reduction in risk with high adherence to the diet. That means that even if you don't follow the MIND diet perfectly, you can still reap the benefits.

All three diets are similar in that they are mostly plant-based, whole-food diets that restrict trans fat and limit saturated fat and refined sugars. However, the MIND diet recommends specific servings of green leafy vegetables and berries, for example, because they contain vitamin E, folate, lutein, beta carotene, and flavonoids, which we know positively impact brain health. The MIND diet also specifies daily and weekly consumption of nuts and seeds, whole grains and starchy vegetables, beans and legumes, seafood, lean poultry, olive oil, fruits, and low-starch vegetables, depending on their nutrient composition and its impact on brain health.

The thing I love most about the MIND diet is how approachable and feasible it is. The diet's modest recommendations on how many servings of the brain-healthy foods you should eat allows you to set attainable goals. For example, foods like fish and berries can be expensive and difficult to find in season, depending on your geographic location and the time of year. If you live in a colder climate, finding fresh berries in the winter is unlikely, or consuming six servings of fish each week can be expensive or not to everyone's taste. The MIND diet recommends just two to three servings of berries per week and just one serving of fatty fish per week, while still reaping the brain-health benefits. As a registered dietitian, I believe that the best kind of diet is one that recommends a wide variety of high-quality, nutritious foods but incorporates them in a realistic, attainable, feasible, and delicious way. After all, as I've been known to say, what good is a diet if you're not going to follow it?

HEALTHY MIND FOODS

MIND-friendly food groups include leafy green vegetables, low-starch vegetables, whole grains and starchy vegetables, beans and legumes, berries, nuts and seeds, seafood, poultry, and vegetable oils. These are not the only foods you'll consume while following the MIND diet, but they should be the ones you consume most often, as they're loaded with brain-healthy nutrients. The food groups listed first are those you should eat daily, followed by the foods you should eat at least weekly.

Leafy Greens

Leafy greens are one of the most important components of the MIND diet because they are rich in vitamin E, folate, lutein, and beta carotene, which are four of the key brain-healthy nutrients outlined in the MIND diet. Leafy greens include arugula, spinach, kale, romaine lettuce, mustard greens, Swiss and rainbow chard, turnip and beet greens, Napa cabbage, watercress, and spring mix. Based on the 2012 Rush Memory Aging Project, we should consume one serving of leafy greens each day. And while that may seem like a lofty goal, greens are one of the easiest ingredients to add to a wide variety of dishes, such as casseroles, soups, stews, smoothies, pasta dishes, burgers, and tacos, and of course, are the perfect base to any salad. In most of my recipes I suggest spinach or kale, as they're the most common of the leafy green vegetables, but feel free to swap them out for one of the more robust greens, like beet greens or Swiss chard.

Serving recommendations: 1 or more servings per day of leafy green vegetables
Serving size: 1 cup raw or ½ cup cooked leafy green vegetables

Low-Starch Vegetables

Low-starch veggies are naturally low in calories and saturated fat and loaded with fiber, vitamins, minerals, and antioxidants. Because of this, it's nearly impossible to overconsume vegetables, and most of us don't consume enough. The MIND diet recommends eating just one serving per day to benefit brain health! While one serving a day is a great place to start, I encourage you to enjoy vegetables with every meal. There are multiple ways to incorporate more vegetables into your diet, and to make them taste delicious. Roast vegetables and serve them as a side or the base of a breakfast hash, add grated vegetables to baked goods, and include at least a handful in casseroles, soups, and sauces.

Serving recommendations: 1 or more servings per day of low-starch vegetables
Serving size: 1 cup raw or ½ cup cooked vegetables

Starchy Vegetables and Whole Grains

The MIND diet doesn't suggest avoiding carbs altogether, but instead it suggests that you choose the most fiber- and nutrient-dense versions available. Potatoes, yams, corn, winter squash, peas, brown rice, whole-grain bread, whole-grain pasta, barley, wheat berries, kamut, farro, bulgur, corn, oats, rye, teff, spelt, and sorghum plus pseudo grains like quinoa, amaranth, millet, buckwheat, and wild rice are MIND-approved. They are rich in B vitamins and are a moderate source of vitamin E, both of which support cognitive function. Be sure to check the ingredients list and choose products made with 100 percent whole grains or those which simply list the grain as the only ingredient, such as "brown rice."

Serving recommendations: 3 servings or more per day of whole grains or starchy vegetables
Serving size: 1 slice whole-grain bread, ½ cup brown rice or peas, 1 medium-size potato or sweet potato

Berries

Berries are a great source of fiber, vitamins, minerals, and antioxidants and are included as a weekly food in the MIND diet because of their flavonoid content. A 2019 study in *Journals of Gerontology* found that eating blueberries may preserve cognitive ability and reverse some age-related cognitive deficits. We also know from research that those who consume more berries have slower rates of cognitive decline than those who consume berries less often. It's safe to say that berries play an important role in preserving cognition and they're also delicious and versatile.

They make the perfect topping for pancakes, waffles, yogurt, or oatmeal; a base for smoothies; and a featured ingredient in a leafy green salad or dessert.

Serving recommendations: 2 or more servings per week of berries

Serving size: ½ cup raw or frozen berries

SUPER NUTRIENTS TO KNOW

In addition to the brain-healthy nutrients we discussed earlier, there are a few others that may be linked to reduced risk of cognitive decline.

Choline. A key nutrient for regulating memory and mood and synthesizing DNA, choline is essential for optimal brain function. A study in the *American Journal of Clinical Nutrition* showed a relationship between higher choline intake and better cognitive performance. Choline is found in eggs, salmon, cod, cauliflower, broccoli, and beef and chicken livers.

Vitamin D. While more research regarding the relationship between vitamin D and brain health is necessary, a 2017 study in *Alzheimer's and Dementia* concluded that study participants who were deficient in vitamin D exhibited a faster rate of cognitive decline than those with normal vitamin D levels. Low vitamin D levels may also contribute to depressive symptoms and increase risk of depression, according to a 2017 study in the journal *Neuropsychiatry*. Vitamin D is found in cod liver oil; fish like tuna, salmon, sardines, and swordfish; milk and yogurt; fortified orange juice and cereals; and eggs.

Cannabis. Although research is limited, some studies show medical cannabis in whole-plant, extract form may be an effective treatment for cognitive impairment. The jury is still out on whether medical cannabis may help reduce risk of cognitive decline.

Nuts and Seeds

Nuts and seeds are packed with nutrients, including B vitamins, vitamin E, healthy fats, and minerals. Each nut and seed has a unique nutrient profile, but overall, it's their antioxidant and anti-inflammatory properties that make them good for brain health. Research shows that nut intake is associated with better cognition, and walnut consumption in particular is associated with better memory scores. This could be because walnuts have more omega-3 fatty acids than other nuts. However, the MIND diet recommends consuming a variety of nuts, including almonds, cashews, pecans, pistachios, macadamia nuts, walnuts, Brazil nuts, and peanuts—also, sunflower, pumpkin, and sesame seeds. They are a filling snack, provide crunch to multiple types of dishes, and add texture and flavor to desserts.

Serving recommendations: 5 or more servings per week of nuts
Serving size: 1 ounce nuts or seeds, 1 tablespoon nut or seed butter

Seafood

One of the few food sources of DHA, seafood contains the type of omega-3 that can protect from the effects of oxidative stress on the brain. Most types of seafood contain DHA, but these fatty varieties contain the most: salmon, herring, mackerel, tuna, sardines, rainbow trout, oysters, and mussels. Clams, crab, lobster, squid, scallops, shrimp, Alaskan pollock, rockfish, snapper, grouper, flounder, sole, halibut, ocean perch, cod, haddock, tilapia, catfish, mahi mahi, orange roughy, and imitation crab also contain omega-3s. Consuming just one serving of seafood rich in omega-3 per week can lead to a positive impact on brain health, according to MIND diet research. However, if you enjoy fish and shellfish, feel free to consume them more than once a week. Broiling, baking, roasting, poaching, and sautéing are just a few of the ways to prepare fish and seafood.

Serving recommendations: 1 or more servings per week of seafood
Serving size: 3 to 4 ounces of fish or shellfish

Poultry

Chicken and turkey are quite popular in cooking because they're mild tasting, affordable, and versatile. Poultry is a great source of B vitamins, which is one of the key MIND diet nutrients. The breast and wings are considered lean and are often referred to as white meat. Poultry skin and meat from the thighs and legs, referred to as dark meat, are high in saturated fat. This doesn't mean you can't enjoy them sometimes, but I recommend eating the leaner cuts more often. Boneless, skinless cooked chicken breasts can be added to soups, salads, casseroles, burrito bowls, and tacos. I recommend marinating them or rubbing them with spices and grilling, sautéing, or roasting them. No matter how you cook poultry, cooking it properly can prevent it from drying out; use an instant-read thermometer and cook poultry to 165°F for best results.

Serving recommendations: 2 or more servings per week of lean poultry
Serving size: 3 to 4 ounces of lean poultry

Beans and Legumes

Beans and legumes are a cost-effective way to beef up your diet with B vitamins, protein, and fiber. They are easy to prepare and can be added to almost everything we eat. Bean varieties include light and dark red kidney, cannellini, great northern, pinto, and black beans. Lentils, chickpeas, lima beans, peas, and soybeans, including edamame and tofu, are all legumes, which are MIND-friendly foods. If using canned beans or legumes, look for the low-sodium or no-added-salt varieties so you're in control of how much salt you put in the dish. I make beans and legumes the star of many dishes, including soups, stews, chilis, casseroles, curries, and tacos.

Serving recommendations: 3 or more servings per week of beans and legumes
Serving size: ½ cup cooked beans or legumes

Oils

There are an overwhelming number of oil options at the supermarket, and not surprisingly, each is marketed as the best oil for your culinary needs, making it all the more difficult to decide which oil to use and when. Extra-virgin olive oil is most recommended for use with the MIND diet because it contains mostly monounsaturated fats, vitamin E, and antioxidants. Extra-virgin olive oil should not be used for high-heat cooking like grilling and roasting because it has a low smoke point, meaning it burns easily. For this reason, extra-virgin olive oil is the best choice for low or medium-heat cooking, such as for making salad dressings or sautéing. For high-heat cooking, I use avocado oil, as it has a high smoke point and is mostly made up of monounsaturated fats like extra-virgin olive oil. There are a wide variety of other vegetable oils that are great for cooking, but extra-virgin olive oil and avocado oil are among the most nutritious. Other specialty oils, like sesame and walnut, can be used to flavor dishes right before serving. I occasionally use coconut oil for baking, but don't recommend it as an everyday cooking oil.

Serving recommendations: Use as your main cooking oil
Serving size: 1 tablespoon oil

FOOD AND MOOD

While we've heavily discussed nutrition and its relationship to cognition and neurodegenerative diseases, as there is strong evidence to link the two, it is also important to note that some recent studies show a link between diet and mood disorders. A 2019 review in *Molecular Psychiatry* concluded that following the Mediterranean diet provides some protection against depression. A 2019 study in *Public Library of Science* showed that a healthy diet rich in fruits, vegetables, fish, and lean meat is associated with reduced risk of depression.

INGREDIENTS TO LIMIT

I am not a fan of restriction and I do believe that the cornerstone of a healthy diet and of having a good relationship with food is feeling free to consume the foods you enjoy eating. However, it is important to note that some foods, when consumed in excess, are not going to do your health any favors. That's why it's important to understand the research-backed MIND diet recommendations and use them to develop a balanced plan so you can be successful in reaching your health goals *while* enjoying what you eat. (Yes, these are not mutually exclusive!) The important thing to remember is that consuming small amounts of these "sometimes foods" will likely not increase your risk of cognitive decline or cardiovascular diseases. I will show you how to enjoy these foods in moderation in the recipe section.

Red Meat

The saturated fat content of red meat is what lands it on this list, even though it is a good source of B_{12} and iron. The Dietary Guidelines for Americans suggests consuming no more than 10 percent of your calories from saturated fat (or less than 20 grams per day), and the MIND diet suggests limiting red meat consumption to no more than three servings of red meat per week. There is no direct research connecting cognitive decline with the consumption of red meat, but we do know that excessive saturated fat intake can increase your risk for cardiovascular diseases, which can impact brain function. This does not mean that you need to cut out red meat entirely. However, if you eat red meat daily, I'd suggest replacing a few of those meals with seafood, poultry, or a meatless meal. Also, be sure to choose lean red meat cuts like tenderloin, sirloin, and top round when you do serve red meat. Some studies show that grass-fed beef can have up to five times as much omega-3 and may have more beta carotene than grain-fed beef, but grain-fed beef has more monounsaturated fatty acids than grass-fed. When planning your meals, you can use this information to make an informed decision on whether to choose grass- or grain-fed beef.

Serving recommendations: 3 or fewer servings per week of beef, pork, or lamb
Serving size: 3 ounces for women; 5 ounces for men

Whole-Fat Dairy

Like red meat, butter, cream, and cheese are high in saturated fat. I suggest using these in small amounts as an enhancement to a dish instead of as the main ingredient. For richness and flavor, I like to sprinkle Parmesan or feta cheese on casseroles and salads, and finish soups with a few tablespoons of cream. I recommend baking with oil and occasionally butter, rather than margarine or shortening, as they contain trans fats.

Serving recommendations: 1 serving of butter per day; 1 serving or less of cheese per week
Serving size: 1 tablespoon butter; 1 ounce cheese

AVOIDING TRANS FATS

Trans fats, labeled as hydrogenated oils, are linked to increased risk of cardiovascular diseases. When it comes to fats, it's recommended to consume mono- and polyunsaturated fats most often, saturated fats sometimes, and to eliminate trans fats from your diet or consume them very rarely. Trans fats are found in foods like vegetable shortening and margarine, deep-fried foods, some coffee creamers, baked goods, and some packaged snacks like crackers. Avoid cooking or baking with shortening and margarine and avoid packaged foods with partially or fully hydrogenated oils listed as an ingredient. Instead, cook with olive and avocado oils most often and use real butter in moderation.

Fried Food

Deep-fried foods such as French fries and donuts are high in trans fats. A 2003 study in *Archives of Neurology* concluded that the consumption of trans fatty acids may increase risk of Alzheimer's disease. More research is needed on how trans fat intake relates to brain health, but we do know that a high intake of saturated and trans fats—especially trans fat—is linked to increased risk of cardiovascular diseases. In addition, deep-fried foods in general do not provide much nutrition in comparison to other brain-health-promoting foods, so limit them to one serving or less per week.

Serving recommendations: 1 serving or less per week

Serving size: 1 donut; 1 small order of French fries

Sweets

Sweets and pastries are typically high in sugar as well as saturated and trans fats, and rarely provide much nutritional value. The MIND diet recommends limiting sweets and pastries to five servings or less per week and to focus more on consuming foods that are packed with brain-supportive nutrients. I do believe that it's important to include foods in your diet that you enjoy, such as chocolate chip cookies, but it's important to be strategic about it. I've included a handful of dessert recipes that feature MIND-friendly foods which should also satisfy your sweet tooth.

Serving recommendations: Fewer than 5 servings per week

Serving size: 1 cookie; 1 piece of cake or pie; 1 cupcake

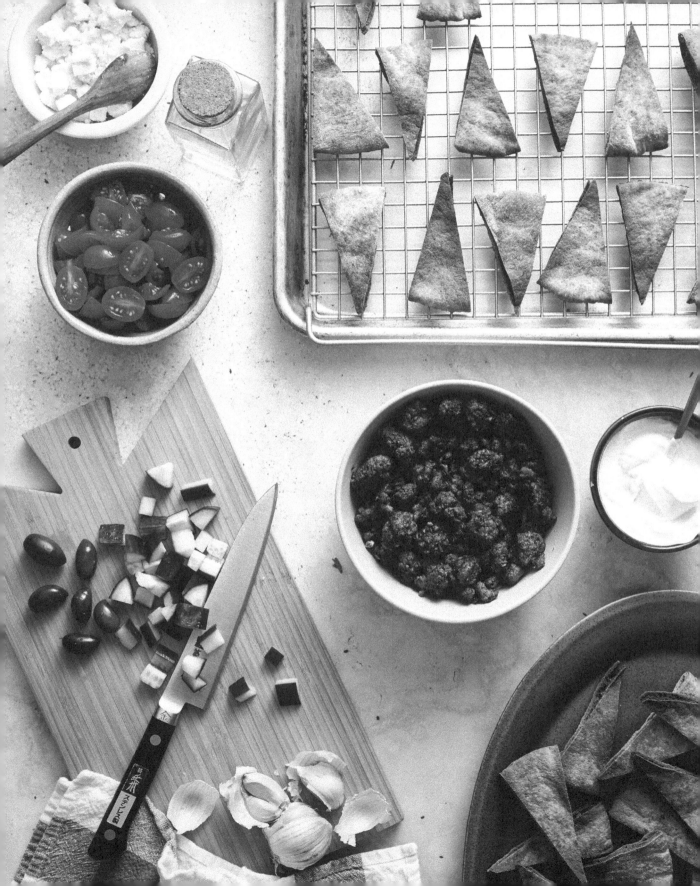

CHAPTER THREE

A Brain-Healthy Life

Now that we've covered the basics of the MIND diet, it's time to put it into practice—this is the fun (and delicious) part! That means we're going to cook and eat our way to better health and improved cognition. I've put together 75 scrumptious recipes that feature MIND diet foods and have shared tips on how to reach the MIND diet recommendations on a daily basis. You will also see pantry, refrigerator, and freezer must-have lists; tips for flavoring your dishes with herbs and spices; and simple ways to live a brain-healthy lifestyle.

SETTING THE STAGE FOR YOUR MIND DIET

By following the MIND diet guidelines, you can reduce your risk of developing Alzheimer's disease and dementia by up to 53 percent! By incorporating more brain-supportive nutrients into your diet, you may also see improvements in brain efficiency, energy levels, and mood. And while adopting new eating habits may seem a little overwhelming at first, once you get the hang of it, eating more MIND-friendly foods should become second nature. After all, this type of eating pattern is not a "diet" in the traditional sense. It's simply about incorporating more nutrient-dense foods into your lifestyle and being more mindful of your portion sizes for the "sometimes foods." Remember that I am here to help you learn to cook with brain-healthy ingredients in simple ways so you can reap the health benefits long-term.

It's also important to note that your diet as a whole is important for reducing your risk of metabolic syndrome and other chronic conditions, so consider evaluating an appropriate number of calories and macronutrients (carbs, protein, and fats) for your specific needs to maintain a healthy weight and help support your overall health. Determining your specific nutrition needs can also help optimize your energy levels.

When you start thumbing through the recipes, you'll notice many ingredients are prefaced by green arrows—those are the MIND diet-specific foods. My goal is to incorporate several of these foods into each recipe to not only help you reach your goals, but to show you how versatile the ingredients are. I hope once you eat your way through this book, you'll be able to apply those same tips and tricks in your own recipes. But before we dive into the recipes, there are some other things you can do to live a brain-healthy life that aren't related to what you put on your plate.

BRAIN-HEALTHY HABITS

While proper nutrition is a powerful tool in reducing risk of cognitive decline, lifestyle habits such as regular exercise, adequate sleep and hydration, stress management techniques, and intellectual pursuits can also preserve cognition. These are the puzzle pieces that impact your overall health and are just as important as diet. Perhaps you exercise a few times a week or have little trouble drinking enough water, and that's great! But if there is an area that you feel could be improved, start by setting a small goal and working on it.

Exercise

Research shows that regular aerobic exercise, such as walking, biking, running, and swimming, is protective of both brain function and cardiovascular health. A 2011 review in the Mayo Clinic Proceedings suggests regular moderate-intensity exercise should be considered a "prescription" for preserving cognition and reducing risk of Alzheimer's disease and dementia. To fend off chronic disease, the National Institutes of Health suggests at least 2 hours and 30 minutes per week, or 30 minutes per day, of moderate-intensity aerobic exercise for adults. Regular exercise may also help improve mood and energy levels. A 2018 review in Exercise and Sport Sciences Reviews concluded that regular physical activity can reduce tension, depressive symptoms, and anger and improve energy. Research shows resistance and strength training can build muscle, maintain healthy bones, and improve coordination, and recent studies show it can reduce depressive symptoms and significantly improve cognitive function, according to the Journal of the American Medical Association Psychiatry and the Journal of the American Geriatrics Society. I recommend including resistance and strength training exercises in your exercise routine at least one to two times per week.

Sleep

There are a few mechanisms that link sleep with brain health. The first may be the relationship between sleep and toxin removal in the brain. Researchers believe that brain waves and electrical signals during sleep may remove toxins from the brain that are associated with neurodegenerative disease, according to a 2019 study in Science. The second may be the relationship between aging and age-related diseases. Good sleep becomes harder to maintain as you age and the prevalence of sleep disorders increases with age, as more people are likely to take medication that can disturb sleep. A 2014 review in Nature Reviews Neurology suggested a correlation between sleep deprivation and Alzheimer's. Sleep deprivation increases the concentration of amyloid peptides in the brain, which can lead to the development of Alzheimer's disease, while getting the recommended amount of sleep has the opposite effect. Sleep apnea, a common condition that can deprive your body of oxygen and have harmful effects on brain tissue, is common in older adults and those with cardiovascular diseases and obesity. Because it's more difficult to maintain healthy sleep patterns as you get older, you may have to change up your routine and habits in order to get enough sleep. The National Institute on Aging recommends that adults get seven to nine hours of sleep every night. To achieve that, it's important to set a regular sleep schedule, avoid late-afternoon napping, avoid caffeine in the afternoon and evening, avoid large meals before bedtime, turn TV and cell phone screens off 30 minutes before bed, and keep your bedroom at a comfortable temperature to give your brain and body the opportunity to rest and reset. If you suffer from insomnia, I recommend that you talk with your doctor.

Mood

Having a positive outlook on life has been linked to cognitive preservation. A 2012 study in the Archives in General Psychiatry reported a reduced risk of Alzheimer's disease and improved cognitive function in those study participants who reported higher levels of purpose in life. A study done at Rush University Medical Center showed that those who had a strong sense of purpose—who felt they had goals in life, a sense of direction, and felt good about their past accomplishments and their outlook for the future—scored higher on memory and thinking tests. Researchers believe that this may be because they have high cognitive reserve, or an enhanced network of connections between brain cells that preserves their memory and thinking skills. It's easier said than done, but reframing negative thoughts into positive ones, such as through a gratitude journal, can improve your overall health, and specifically, brain health.

Stress Relief

While it's no surprise that having the ability to manage stress is a valuable life skill and can contribute to improved health, we also know high stress levels can increase risk for cognitive decline. A 2003 study in Neurology concluded that the risk of developing Alzheimer's disease was doubled in participants with higher levels of psychological distress compared to those with lower levels of psychological distress.

A 2019 review in the Journal of Neural Transmission notes stress as a risk factor for Alzheimer's disease and explains that anxiety may also increase risk. Activities like exercising regularly; engaging in relaxing activities such as yoga, meditation, or reading; and talking to a loved one or friend can provide stress relief and improve your health. If negative thoughts and stress become out of control and are impacting your day-to-day life, I suggest that you seek professional help.

Mindfulness

Mindfulness is a type of meditation that helps you focus on being intensely aware of what you're sensing and feeling in the moment and often involves breathing and relaxation techniques, as well as guided imagery. The practice of mindfulness may improve mental functioning while reducing stress, symptoms of anxiety and depression, insomnia, and high blood pressure, all of which have been linked to cognition and the risk of neurodegenerative diseases. A 2011 study in Psychiatry Research suggested that participation in the Mindfulness-Based Stress Reduction (MBSR) program was associated with changes in gray matter concentration in the brain regions involved in learning, memory, and emotions. If you're interested in learning more about mindfulness practices, search for a MBSR class in your area or check out calm.com for free mindfulness resources.

Intellectually Stimulating Pursuits

Reading books, playing word games, and learning to play an instrument are all intellectually stimulating activities that can impact cognition. Studies also show that you can preserve cognitive function by having a healthy social life and surrounding yourself with people you enjoy spending time with. Some studies have shown that participation in leisure activities that require memory and reasoning skills, like chess and bridge, are protective of cognition. A review in the Journal of Psychosocial Nursing and Mental Health Services concluded that social integration, engagement with family, and participating in community activities were protective of cognitive abilities. However, studies also show that frequent negative social interactions can result in lower levels of cognition. The moral of the story is to participate in a range of mentally stimulating activities and maintain a positive social life.

Good Hydration

Water is necessary in nearly every function in the human body, making adequate hydration crucial for maintaining good health. Water is instrumental in helping the kidneys and liver flush out waste products and helping dissolve nutrients so they're easily accessible to the body. Water also plays a critical role in delivering nutrients to the brain and protecting organs and tissue. Some studies show that being dehydrated may impair brain function and cause low energy levels. It's important to recognize that if you feel thirsty, you're already dehydrated. The Mayo Clinic recommends drinking at least eight glasses a day, although depending on factors such as your weight, height, and activity level, you may need more. A few ways to achieve drinking at least 64 ounces of water every day is to keep a refillable water bottle at home and work, and to eat foods with a high water content, like fruits and vegetables. To measure your hydration status, check your urine color; colorless or light yellow urine generally means you're well-hydrated.

BRAIN FOOD BY THE SEASONS

Vegetables and fruits are plentiful in the MIND diet, so it's important to understand their seasonality and the different varieties available to us. Fresh fruits and vegetables are generally the most popular for cooking, and when they're in season, are affordable and of good quality. Produce like apples, avocados, bananas, lemons, limes, garlic, carrots, and celery are available year-round and are easy to find. When fruits and veggies aren't in season, frozen, canned, and dried are also an option. Frozen fruits and vegetables are generally just as (if not more) nutritious as fresh, as they're picked at their peak of freshness and flash frozen to preserve quality and nutrition. Canned and dried fruits and vegetables are also nourishing, but be sure to check the nutrition label to avoid added sugar or salt. Follow along with this seasonality guide to help you choose a wide variety of produce throughout the year.

Spring

- Apricots
- Asparagus
- Broccoli
- Collard greens
- Garlic
- Kale
- Kiwis
- Lettuce
- Mushrooms
- Onions
- Peas
- Radishes
- Rhubarb
- Spinach
- Strawberries
- Swiss chard
- Turnips

Summer

- Beets
- Bell peppers
- Blackberries
- Blueberries
- Cantaloupe
- Cherries
- Corn
- Cucumbers
- Eggplant
- Green beans
- Honeydew melons
- Lima beans
- Mangos
- Okra
- Peaches
- Plums
- Raspberries
- Strawberries
- Summer squash
- Tomatillos
- Tomatoes
- Watermelon
- Wax beans
- Zucchini

Fall

- Beets
- Bell peppers
- Broccoli
- Brussels sprouts
- Cabbage
- Cauliflower
- Collard greens
- Cranberries
- Ginger
- Grapes
- Green beans
- Kale
- Kiwis
- Lettuce
- Mangos
- Mushrooms
- Onions
- Parsnips
- Pears

- Peas
- Potatoes
- Pumpkins
- Radishes
- Raspberries
- Rutabagas
- Spinach
- Sweet potatoes and yams
- Swiss chard
- Turnips
- Winter squash

Winter

- Beets
- Brussels sprouts
- Cabbage
- Collard greens
- Grapefruit
- Kale

- Kiwis
- Leeks
- Onions
- Oranges
- Parsnips
- Pears
- Potatoes
- Pumpkins
- Rutabagas
- Sweet potatoes and yams
- Swiss chard
- Turnips
- Winter squash

YOUR BRAIN ON ALCOHOL

Studies show that consuming alcohol in moderation can protect your heart and your brain. In a 2012 review in *Frontiers in Bioscience*, researchers found lower risks of cognitive decline and dementia in light to moderate drinkers compared with people who never drink or excessively consume. Multiple studies show that moderate wine consumption can produce a reduction in cardiovascular and neurodegenerative mortality. Resveratrol, a compound contained in red wine that has antioxidant properties, is the reason for the link between wine consumption and health. The MIND diet recommends consuming no more than one 5-ounce glass of wine per day, but that doesn't mean that if you're a nondrinker you need to start drinking to be healthy. Also, alcohol can be addictive. If you have a personal or family history of alcoholism, abstinence is best. It's wise to discuss alcohol intake with your doctor.

PANTRY, REFRIGERATOR, AND FREEZER STAPLES

Cooking and meal planning can become more efficient and easier when you have your pantry, refrigerator, and freezer stocked with a few staples. I've compiled a list of some of the items you'll use regularly in the recipes throughout this book, ranging from components of well-balanced meals to condiments, seasonings, and sauces that provide flavor or give a boost of nutrition. You don't need to purchase every single item on the list, but I recommend starting with a good base of oils, spices, vinegars, canned or dried beans and lentils, canned tomatoes, aromatics like onions and garlic, and frozen vegetables, fruits, and meats.

Pantry Staples

Oils and Vinegars

- Apple cider vinegar
- Avocado oil
- Balsamic vinegar
- Coconut oil
- Cooking spray
- Extra-virgin olive oil
- Red wine vinegar
- Rice wine vinegar
- Sesame oil
- White wine vinegar

Herbs and Spices

- Bay leaves
- Celery seeds
- Chili powder
- Dried dill
- Dried oregano leaves
- Dried sage
- Garam masala
- Garlic powder
- Ground black pepper
- Ground cayenne pepper
- Ground cinnamon
- Ground cumin
- Ground ginger
- Ground mustard powder
- Ground nutmeg
- Italian seasoning
- Kosher or sea salt
- Onion powder
- Red pepper flakes
- Smoked paprika

Nuts, Seeds, and Grains

- Brown rice
- Chia seeds
- Ground flaxseed
- Nuts (walnuts, almonds, peanuts, cashews, pine nuts, pecans, etc.)
- Panko bread crumbs
- Quinoa
- Seeds (sunflower, sesame, pumpkin, etc.)

Baking Supplies

- All-purpose flour
- Baking powder
- Baking soda
- Cornmeal
- Cornstarch
- Dark chocolate chips
- Old-fashioned rolled oats
- Raisins
- Unsweetened shredded coconut
- Vanilla extract
- Wheat or oat bran
- Whole-wheat or oat flour

Canned Goods

- Beans (black beans, chickpeas, cannellini, lentils, etc.)
- Crushed tomatoes
- Diced tomatoes
- Low-sodium bouillon
- Nut or seed butters
- Stock or broth (vegetable, chicken, beef)
- Tomato paste

Sweeteners

- Dark brown sugar
- Granulated sugar
- Honey

Refrigerator Staples

- Butter
- Dark leafy greens
- Dijon mustard
- Ketchup
- Maple syrup
- Mayonnaise
- Salad greens
- Sriracha
- Worcestershire sauce
- Yellow mustard

Freezer Staples

- Assorted fruit
- Assorted vegetables
- Beef
- Berries
- Dark leafy greens
- Fish and seafood
- Pork
- Poultry

SMART FLAVORS

One of the easiest ways to add flavor to food in a healthy way is with herbs and spices. They add immense and unique flavor to dishes and can be combined in fun ways to change things up. In conjunction with acidic ingredients like citrus juice and vinegars, we can spice up a dish without having to add as much salt. Yes, you will find salt in the recipes in this book because herbs, spices, and acidic ingredients do not completely eliminate the need for salt. Instead, they just help reduce the amount needed while still achieving delicious-tasting food. It is important to note that you can modify the amount of salt you add to your recipes. The amount suggested in my recipes is just that—a suggestion.

Many herbs and spices have antioxidant and anti-inflammatory properties and have been used for medicinal purposes for hundreds of years. According to Harvard University, cinnamon, cloves, ginger, sage, turmeric, and cardamom, to name a few, may reduce inflammation, improve memory, increase attention, boost mood, and lower blood pressure. While the MIND diet doesn't provide specific recommendations for the dosage of each herb and spice, I encourage you to use a variety in all your recipes.

You also may be wondering what to use if you want to sweeten your coffee, tea, and smoothies. I prefer to use a small amount of regular sugar or stevia. As you'll see throughout the recipe section, I tend to use maple syrup or honey, and occasionally granulated or dark brown sugar, to make baked goods and desserts palatable. A small amount of added sugar won't hurt; just be careful not to go overboard.

BRAIN FOOD TRACKER

MIND Food	Monday	Tuesday	Wednesday
Leafy greens (Suggested: at least 1 serving per day)			
Low-starch vegetables (Suggested: at least 1 serving per day)			
Starchy vegetables/ whole grains (Suggested: at least 3 servings per day)			
Berries (Suggested: at least 2 servings per week)			
Nuts and seeds (Suggested: at least 5 servings per week)			
Seafood (Suggested: at least 1 serving per week)			
Poultry (Suggested: at least 2 servings per week)			
Beans and legumes (Suggested: at least 3 servings per week)			
Oils (Suggested: Use olive oil or avocado oil as your main cooking oils)			

Thursday	Friday	Saturday	Sunday	Total

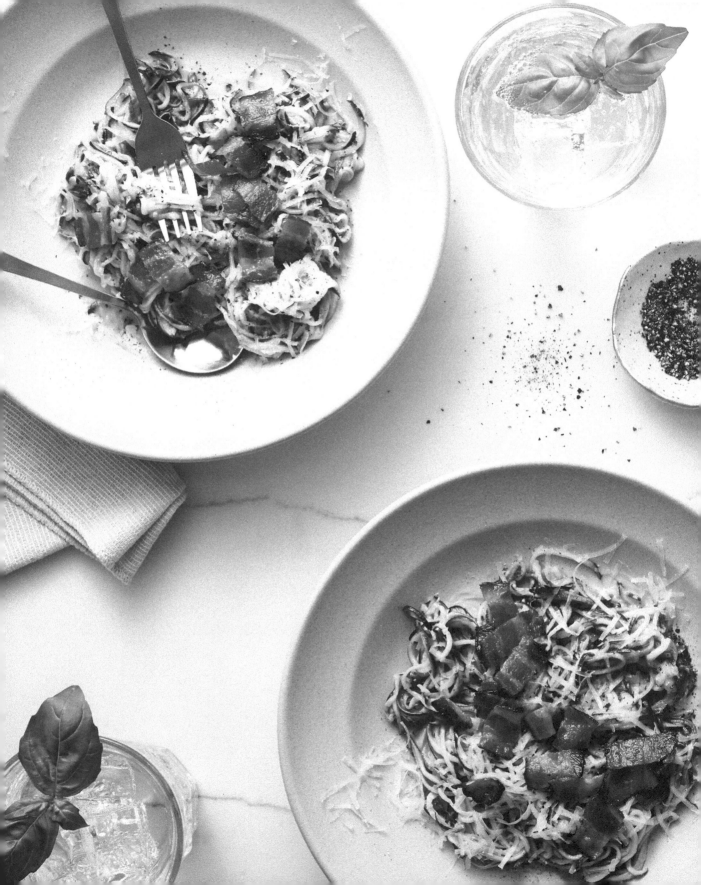

THE RECIPES

The exciting part is getting into the kitchen and putting your MIND diet knowledge to work! The recipes in the following chapters are packed with brain-healthy foods and other nourishing ingredients that are designed to help you meet the recommendations of the MIND diet and eat a balanced diet overall. They are also balanced with complex carbs and fiber, protein, and heart-healthy fats to help reduce your risk of developing chronic conditions and maintain focus and energy levels throughout the day.

I've included tips with each recipe, including variation tips on how to keep things interesting, substitution tips for special diets, and cooking tips for ways to make your recipes extra delicious. Please note that for any recipes that call for milk, I used nonfat milk, but you can choose whatever milk you prefer. MIND diet-specific ingredients are prefaced with a green arrow. Remember that not every ingredient you use is a MIND diet "superfood," and that's okay! My goal is to help you to incorporate more nourishing foods into your diet to help preserve cognition in a delicious way.

Smashed Avocado Toast with Poached Eggs, Page 48

CHAPTER FOUR
Breakfast

Wild Berry Cashew Smoothie

Smoothies are a simple and delicious way to pack loads of MIND diet foods into one meal. Ingredients like berries, leafy greens, and nuts make the perfect base for a nutritious breakfast or snack when whirled together with milk or yogurt. You can spice up your smoothie with cinnamon, ginger, and turmeric and add a boost of omega-3s and fiber with flax or chia seeds.

1¾ cups milk

▶ ¼ cup unsalted cashews

▶ 1½ cups frozen mixed berries

▶ 1 cup baby spinach leaves or chopped kale

1 medium frozen banana, peeled

▶ 2 tablespoons ground flaxseed

GLUTEN-FREE
VEGETARIAN

Serves: 2

Prep Time: 5 to 10 minutes

Substitution tip
Use cow's, almond, coconut, rice, cashew, or soy milk.

Variation tip
Try frozen peaches, pineapple, or mango instead of berries. Add a scoop of vanilla or unflavored protein powder to keep you full until lunchtime.

1. Pour the milk and cashews into a blender. Let sit for 5 minutes.

2. Add the berries, spinach, banana, and flaxseed to the blender. Purée until very smooth. Serve immediately.

3. It is not recommended to make smoothies in advance.

Per Serving: Calories: 298; Total fat: 15g; Saturated fat: 2g; Cholesterol: 0mg; Sodium: 136mg; Carbohydrates: 37g; Fiber: 7g; Sugar: 18g; Protein: 7g

Apple-Cinnamon Bran Muffins

Bran is one of three parts of a wheat kernel that is a great source of fiber, protein, B vitamins, and minerals. Paired with apples, walnuts, vanilla, and a touch of brown sugar, these bran muffins are a wholesome, satisfying, and brain-healthy way to snack.

- 1½ cups wheat or oat bran
- 1 cup whole-wheat or oat flour

  2 teaspoons ground cinnamon

  1 teaspoon baking powder

  1 teaspoon baking soda

  ½ teaspoon kosher or sea salt
- ⅓ cup avocado oil

  ⅓ cup dark brown sugar
- 1 large egg

  1¼ cups milk

  2 teaspoons pure vanilla extract
- 2 medium firm apples, diced
- ½ cup chopped walnuts or pecans, divided

VEGETARIAN

Makes 12 muffins
Prep Time: 10 to 15 minutes
Cook Time: 20 to 25 minutes

Substitution tip
For gluten-free muffins, omit the bran and wheat flour and use 2½ cups of gluten-free, all-purpose flour instead.

Cooking tip
The trick to a tender muffin is to not overmix the batter. Only stir until ingredients are just combined, and gently fold in the apples and walnuts without over-stirring.

1. Preheat the oven to 350°F. Line a 12-cup muffin tin with liners. Set aside.

2. In a mixing bowl, whisk together the bran, flour, cinnamon, baking powder, baking soda, and salt.

3. In another mixing bowl, whisk together the oil and brown sugar until fluffy. Whisk in the egg until incorporated. Whisk in the milk and vanilla extract. Pour the wet mixture into the dry ingredients and mix together with a spatula until just combined. Fold in the apples and ¼ cup of walnuts.

4. Scoop the muffin batter into the muffin cups, filling the batter to just below the top of the muffin liners. Sprinkle each with the remaining ¼ cup of walnuts. Bake for 18 to 22 minutes, or until muffins are just set. Let cool, then serve.

5. The muffins can be prepped in advance and stored in an airtight container or resealable plastic bag for up to 5 days at room temperature.

Per Serving (1 muffin): Calories: 192; Total fat: 11g; Saturated fat: 1g; Cholesterol: 17mg; Sodium: 209mg; Carbohydrates: 23g; Fiber: 6g; Sugar: 10g; Protein: 5g

Lemon-Ricotta Pancakes with Blueberry Compote

These pancakes come together in just a few minutes, but you'll feel as if you're eating at a five-star brunch restaurant. The batter makes light, fluffy, and rich lemony flapjacks, and the blueberry compote requires only three ingredients. It's good enough to eat with a spoon.

FOR THE COMPOTE

▸ 1½ cups fresh or frozen blueberries

▸ Zest and juice of ½ medium lemon (about 1 tablespoon each)

1½ teaspoons granulated sugar

FOR THE PANCAKES

▸ 1¼ cups whole-wheat or oat flour

1 tablespoon granulated sugar

2 teaspoons baking powder

½ teaspoon baking soda

¼ teaspoon kosher or sea salt

1 cup ricotta cheese

▸ 2 large eggs

▸ Zest and juice of 2 medium lemons (about ¼ cup each)

¼ cup milk

▸ 2 tablespoons avocado oil

1 teaspoon pure vanilla extract

NUT-FREE
VEGETARIAN

Serves: 5
Prep Time: 5 to 10 minutes
Cook Time: 15 to 20 minutes

Variation tip
Try strawberries, blackberries, or raspberries instead of blueberries in the compote recipe.

Cooking tip
Once mixed, let the batter sit 5 minutes. It'll make for fluffier pancakes.

1. To make the compote, in a small saucepan, stir together the blueberries, lemon zest and juice, and sugar. Bring to a low simmer for 10 to 15 minutes, stirring occasionally, until slightly thickened. Remove from the heat and set aside.

2. To make the pancakes, in a mixing bowl, stir together the flour, sugar, baking powder, baking soda, and salt.

3. In a separate mixing bowl, whisk together the ricotta cheese and eggs until fluffy. Whisk in the lemon zest and juice, milk, oil, and vanilla extract until combined. Fold in the dry ingredients until blended.

4. Heat a large sauté pan or skillet over medium high. Coat with cooking spray. Working in batches, pour ¼ cup batter into the hot skillet and cook for 2 to 3 minutes per side, until set. Repeat with the remaining batter. Serve the pancakes with blueberry compote.

5. The pancakes can be prepped in advance and stored in a large sealed plastic bag or airtight container up to 4 days in the refrigerator. Reheat the pancakes in the microwave 30 to 60 seconds or until heated through. The blueberry compote can be prepped in advance and stored in an airtight container for up to 4 days in the refrigerator. Reheat the compote in the microwave for 30 to 60 seconds, or until heated through, and serve with pancakes.

Per Serving (2 pancakes): Calories: 277; Total fat: 10g; Saturated fat: 2g; Cholesterol: 86mg; Sodium: 471mg; Carbohydrates: 36g; Fiber: 6g; Sugar: 13g; Protein: 12g

Strawberry-Stuffed Almond Crêpes

Crêpes are thin French pancakes that can be made sweet or savory. This sweet version is made with almond meal and stuffed with nut butter, berries, and almonds. It sounds indulgent, but you'll knock out several MIND diet foods first thing in the morning.

- ½ cup almond meal or almond flour
- 3 large eggs

  1½ teaspoons granulated sugar

  1 teaspoon pure vanilla extract

  ¼ teaspoon ground cinnamon

  ⅛ teaspoon kosher or sea salt
- ¼ cup creamy almond or peanut butter
- 1 pint strawberries, hulled and sliced
- ¼ cup sliced almonds

  2 tablespoons pure maple syrup (optional)

DAIRY-FREE
GLUTEN-FREE
VEGETARIAN

Serves: 4
Prep Time: 5 to 10 minutes
Cook Time: 15 to 20 minutes

Substitution tip
Try whole-wheat flour instead of almond meal or almond flour.

Cooking tip
Add ¼ teaspoon pure almond extract for extra almond flavor. Almond meal and almond flour are the same thing; use them interchangeably.

1. In a mixing bowl, whisk together the almond meal, eggs, sugar, vanilla extract, cinnamon, and salt until smooth.

2. Heat a large sauté pan or skillet over medium-high heat. Coat with cooking spray. Working in batches, pour ¼ cup batter into the hot skillet, tilting the pan to let the batter evenly coat the pan. Cook 1 to 2 minutes per side, until set. Remove and set aside and repeat with the remaining batter.

3. Spread the almond butter on each crêpe and sprinkle a layer of strawberry slices and sliced almonds on half of each one. Fold each in half, then in quarters. Top with maple syrup (if using). Serve immediately.

4. The crêpes can be prepped in advance and stored in a large sealed plastic bag or airtight container for up to 4 days in the refrigerator. Reheat in the microwave for 30 to 60 seconds, or until heated through.

Per Serving (1 crêpe): Calories: 327; Total fat: 24g; Saturated fat: 3g; Cholesterol: 140mg; Sodium: 202mg; Carbohydrates: 17g; Fiber: 5g; Sugar: 8g; Protein: 14g

Peanut Butter and Banana Baked Oatmeal

There's nothing better than a square of warm cinnamon-banana oatmeal swirled with peanut butter and berries. And on top of that, you can make one big batch and warm it up for breakfast all week.

- ▶ 1½ cups old-fashioned rolled oats
- 1½ teaspoons ground cinnamon
- 1 teaspoon baking powder
- ½ teaspoon kosher or sea salt
- 2 ripe bananas, peeled and mashed
- ¾ cup milk

- ▶ ⅓ cup creamy peanut butter
- 5 tablespoons pure maple syrup or honey
- ▶ 1 large egg
- 1½ teaspoons pure vanilla extract
- ▶ 1 cup fresh or frozen blueberries or raspberries

VEGETARIAN

Serves: 8
Prep Time: 10 to 15 minutes
Cook Time: 25 to 30 minutes

Substitution tip
Use quick-cooking oats instead of old-fashioned rolled oats. Use almond butter instead of peanut butter.

Variation tip
Swap in chopped mango or peaches instead of berries.

1. Preheat the oven to 350°F. Fit a piece of parchment paper into an 8-inch-square baking dish, allowing it to slightly hang over the top of the dish. Set aside.

2. In a mixing bowl, stir together the oats, cinnamon, baking powder, and salt.

3. In another mixing bowl, whisk together the bananas, milk, peanut butter, maple syrup, egg, and vanilla extract until well combined. Fold in the dry ingredients until blended.

4. Transfer the mixture to the prepared baking dish. Sprinkle the blueberries on top. Bake for 30 to 35 minutes or until set. Let cool slightly, then lift the parchment paper from the pan and slice into 8 squares. Serve immediately.

5. The oatmeal squares can be prepped in advance and stored in a large sealed plastic bag or airtight container for up to 4 days in the refrigerator. Reheat in the microwave for 30 to 60 seconds, or until heated through.

Per Serving: Calories: 204; Total fat: 7g; Saturated fat: 1g; Cholesterol: 23mg; Sodium: 206mg; Carbohydrates: 32g; Fiber: 4g; Sugar: 15g; Protein: 6g

Smashed Avocado Toast with Poached Eggs

Avocado toast may seem trendy, but there's no denying how absolutely delicious it is. The avocados are mashed with lemon, salt, and pepper, and the poached eggs are cooked until the whites are tender and the yolks are perfectly runny, then it's all served up on crusty whole-grain bread, making for a hearty start to the day.

FOR THE EGGS

1 teaspoon white vinegar

▶ 4 large eggs

¼ teaspoon kosher or sea salt

FOR THE TOAST

▶ 2 medium ripe avocados, pitted and peeled

▶ Zest and juice of 1 medium lemon (about 2 tablespoons each)

¼ teaspoon kosher or sea salt

¼ teaspoon freshly ground black pepper

▶ 4 slices whole-grain bread

DAIRY-FREE
NUT-FREE
VEGETARIAN

Serves: 4

Prep Time: 5 to 10 minutes

Cook Time: 10 to 15 minutes

Substitution tip

For a gluten-free version, use gluten-free bread.

Variation tip

Make over-easy eggs instead of poached eggs. Heat a large nonstick skillet on medium-low heat and coat with cooking spray. Crack eggs into the pan and sprinkle with salt. Cook for 2 to 3 minutes per side, or until egg white is set and yolk is runny.

1. To make the eggs, in a stock pot, pour 8 cups of water and bring to a gentle simmer (160°F to 180°F). Stir in the vinegar. Place a few pieces of paper towel on a plate near the stove.

2. Stir the water a bit to create a whirlpool. Crack one egg into a small bowl, then slowly slide it into the simmering vinegar water. Repeat this process with the remaining eggs. Cook 3 to 5 minutes, or until the egg white is set.

3. Remove the eggs with a slotted spoon and place on the paper towel. Sprinkle with salt.

4. To make the toast, in a bowl, combine the avocados, lemon zest and juice, salt, and pepper and mash with the back of a fork. Taste and adjust seasoning, if necessary.

5. Toast the slices of bread. Spread the mashed avocado on the toast and top each with a poached egg. Serve immediately.

6. The poached eggs can be prepped in advance and stored in an airtight container for up to 4 days in the refrigerator. Reheat in the microwave for 30 to 60 seconds, or until heated through.

7. Store the smashed avocado in an airtight container for up to 3 days in the refrigerator. To keep the mashed avocado from browning, top with a thin layer of water; before using, drain the water off and stir the mashed avocado. Assemble toasts just before eating.

Per Serving: Calories: 293; Total fat: 17g; Saturated fat: 3g; Cholesterol: 186mg; Sodium: 216mg; Carbohydrates: 26g; Fiber: 8g; Sugar: 4g; Protein: 12g

Spinach-Artichoke Breakfast Bake

Spinach and artichoke go together like . . . spinach and artichoke. They're quite possibly the best culinary pair, and in this breakfast bake, they are accentuated with garlic, Italian seasonings, and white cheddar. The Greek yogurt provides body and texture to each square, as well as an extra boost of protein.

- 1 teaspoon extra-virgin olive oil
- 4 cups baby spinach leaves
- 3 garlic cloves, minced
- 10 large eggs
- ½ cup plain Greek yogurt
- 1 tablespoon Italian seasoning
- 1½ teaspoons kosher or sea salt
- 1½ teaspoons onion powder
- ½ teaspoon freshly ground black pepper
- ¼ teaspoon red pepper flakes
- 1½ cups frozen, shredded hash browns
- 1 (12-ounce) can artichoke hearts, drained and chopped
- 1 cup shredded white cheddar

GLUTEN-FREE
NUT-FREE
VEGETARIAN

Serves: 6
Prep Time: 10 to 15 minutes
Cook Time: 30 to 35 minutes

Variation tip
Swap out artichoke hearts for chopped bell pepper.

Substitution tip
Use nondairy yogurt and omit the cheddar to make this recipe dairy-free.

1. Preheat the oven to 350°F. Coat a 13-by-9-inch pan with cooking spray. Set aside.

2. In a large sauté pan or skillet, heat the olive oil over medium heat. Add the spinach and cook for 2 to 3 minutes, or until wilted. Stir in the garlic and sauté for an additional 30 to 60 seconds, until fragrant. Set aside.

3. In a large mixing bowl, whisk together the eggs, Greek yogurt, Italian seasoning, salt, onion powder, pepper, and red pepper flakes until well combined. Fold in the cooked spinach and garlic, hash browns, and chopped artichoke hearts.

4. Transfer the mixture to a baking dish. Top with shredded cheese. Bake 30 to 35 minutes, or until set. Let cool slightly, then cut into 6 squares and serve.

5. The breakfast squares can be prepped in advance and stored in an airtight container for up to 5 days in the refrigerator. Reheat in the microwave for 1 to 2 minutes, or until heated through.

Per Serving: Calories: 239; Total fat: 16g; Saturated fat: 7g; Cholesterol: 331mg; Sodium: 648mg; Carbohydrates: 7g; Fiber: 2g; Sugar: 1g; Protein: 18g

Black Bean Breakfast Enchiladas

Sometimes it can be a struggle to fit veggies in at breakfast, but these enchiladas check all the boxes. We have spinach, bell peppers, and black beans tucked inside egg "tortillas" and topped with salsa and heart-healthy avocado. They're covered with zippy enchilada sauce and a light smattering of ooey gooey Monterey Jack cheese, making for one mouthwatering breakfast.

- 8 large eggs
- ½ teaspoon kosher or sea salt, divided
- ½ teaspoon freshly ground black pepper, divided
- 1 teaspoon avocado oil
- 2 cups baby spinach leaves or chopped kale
- 1 medium bell pepper, diced
- 1 (15-ounce) can no-salt-added black beans, drained and rinsed

- 1 tablespoon chili powder
- ½ cup chopped fresh cilantro
- ½ cup shredded Monterey Jack cheese, divided
- ¾ cup low sodium enchilada sauce
- ½ cup fresh salsa
- 1 medium avocado, peeled, pitted, and diced

GLUTEN-FREE
NUT-FREE
VEGETARIAN

Serves: 6
Prep Time: 20 to 25 minutes
Cook Time: 15 to 20 minutes

Cooking tip
If you make your own enchilada sauce, you can control how much salt you add to it. Canned enchilada sauce tends to have a high sodium content.

Variation tip
Try pinto beans instead of black beans.

1. Preheat the oven to 350°F. Coat a 13-by-9-inch pan with cooking spray. Set aside.
2. In a medium mixing bowl, beat the eggs together with ¼ teaspoon salt and ¼ teaspoon pepper.
3. Heat a medium, nonstick sauté pan or skillet over medium heat. To make the "tortillas," coat the pan with cooking spray and add ¼ cup egg mixture to it. Cover and cook for 2 to 3 minutes, until set. Transfer to a cutting board and repeat with the remaining egg mixture.

4. In the same skillet, heat the oil over medium heat. Add the spinach, bell pepper, and black beans and cook for 4 to 5 minutes, or until the pepper is soft. Use the back of a spatula to smash some of the beans. Season with the chili powder and the remaining ¼ teaspoon salt and ¼ teaspoon pepper and stir in the cilantro. Taste and adjust seasoning, if necessary.

5. Scoop black bean mixture into the middle of each egg tortilla and sprinkle with 1 tablespoon of Monterey Jack cheese. Roll them up like enchiladas and tuck each into the prepared baking pan with the seam side down. Pour the enchilada sauce over them and sprinkle with the remaining 2 tablespoons Monterey Jack cheese. Bake for 10 to 15 minutes, or until the cheese is melted and bubbly. Serve the enchiladas topped with salsa and avocado.

6. The breakfast enchiladas can be prepped in advance and stored in an airtight container for up to 5 days in the refrigerator. Reheat in the microwave for 1 to 2 minutes, or until heated through. Top with salsa and avocado just before serving.

Per Serving (1 enchilada): Calories: 295; Total fat: 18g; Saturated fat: 6g; Cholesterol: 266mg; Sodium: 660mg; Carbohydrates: 16g; Fiber: 6g; Sugar: 4g; Protein: 17g

**Spinach, Walnut, and Goat Cheese Salad
with Raspberry Vinaigrette, Page 61**

CHAPTER FIVE

Salads, Soups, and Sides

Vietnamese-Inspired Spring Roll Salad with Peanut Dressing

I've used this peanut dressing in everything from pad Thai to stir fries to this spring roll salad, and it never disappoints. I often hear "This is the BEST peanut sauce I've ever had!" from many who have tried this recipe, so I'm certain you'll love it. Just be sure you make extra so you can put it on everything.

FOR THE DRESSING

- ⅓ cup creamy peanut butter
- 2 tablespoons low-sodium soy sauce
- 2 tablespoons rice wine vinegar
- Zest and juice of 1 medium lime (about 2 tablespoons)
- 1-inch piece fresh ginger, peeled and finely minced
- 1 tablespoon brown sugar
- 2 teaspoons sesame oil
- ½ teaspoon sriracha (optional)

FOR THE SALAD

- 4 ounces brown rice noodles
- 1 medium bell pepper, thinly sliced
- ½ medium English cucumber, julienned
- 1 cup carrots, peeled and shredded
- ½ cup shredded purple cabbage
- ½ cup chopped fresh cilantro (optional)
- ¼ cup chopped fresh mint (optional)
- ½ cup chopped roasted peanuts (optional)

VEGAN

Serves: 8

Prep Time: 15 to 20 minutes

Cook Time: 8 to 10 minutes

Substitution tip
For a gluten-free salad, use tamari instead of soy sauce.

Variation tip
Add 8 ounces diced, cooked shrimp for added protein.

1. To make the dressing, in a medium bowl, whisk together the peanut butter, soy sauce, rice wine vinegar, lime zest and juice, ginger, brown sugar, sesame oil, and sriracha (if using) until combined. If dressing is thick, thin with a splash of water.

2. To make the salad, bring a pot of water to a boil. Break the rice noodles into 2-inch pieces and drop into the water. Cook for 7 to 8 minutes, until *al dente*. Drain and rinse with cold water.

3. Transfer to a large bowl. Add the bell pepper, cucumber, carrots, and cabbage. Add the cilantro (if using), mint (if using), and peanuts (if using) to the bowl. Toss with the peanut dressing. Refrigerate at least 30 minutes.

4. The spring roll salad can be prepped in advance and stored in an airtight container for up to 3 days in the refrigerator.

Per Serving: Calories: 160; Total fat: 7g; Saturated fat: 1g; Cholesterol: 0mg; Sodium: 178mg; Carbohydrates: 23g; Fiber: 3g; Sugar: 6g; Protein: 5g

Greek Chopped Salad with Creamy Feta Dressing

Traditional Greek salad is served with a lemony vinaigrette dressing, but this version comes with a creamy dressing made from olive oil, garlic, dill, oregano, feta, and a touch of mayonnaise. MIND-friendly recipes don't have to be void of ingredients like butter, cream, and mayonnaise—rather, those ingredients should be used in small amounts to enhance a dish. The focus should be on including large doses of brain-healthy foods.

FOR THE DRESSING

▶ ¼ cup extra-virgin olive oil

3 tablespoons mayonnaise

1 tablespoon white wine vinegar

▶ 2 garlic cloves, peeled and minced

1 teaspoon onion powder

1 teaspoon dried oregano leaves

½ teaspoon dried dill (optional)

¼ teaspoon kosher or sea salt

¼ teaspoon freshly ground black pepper

½ cup crumbled feta cheese

FOR THE SALAD

▶ 3 heads romaine lettuce, shredded (about 6 cups)

▶ 1 medium English cucumber, diced

▶ 1 pint cherry tomatoes, quartered

▶ 1 medium green bell pepper, thinly sliced (optional)

▶ ¼ cup pitted, halved kalamata olives

GLUTEN-FREE

NUT-FREE

VEGETARIAN

Serves: 4

Prep Time: 15 to 20 minutes

Substitution tip
Try the salad with chopped kale instead of romaine.

Variation tip
Top the salad with a cooked salmon fillet or chicken breast for a high-protein meal.

1. To make the dressing, in a medium bowl, whisk together the olive oil, mayonnaise, vinegar, garlic, onion powder, oregano, dill (if using), salt, and pepper. Stir in the feta cheese. Taste and adjust seasoning, if necessary.

2. To make the salad, in a large bowl, toss together the romaine lettuce, cucumber, cherry tomatoes, bell pepper (if using), and kalamata olives. Serve with the creamy feta dressing.

3. The feta dressing can be prepped in advance and stored in a separate airtight container for up to 3 days in the refrigerator. The Greek salad can be prepped in advance and stored in airtight containers for up to 3 days in the refrigerator. Drizzle salad with dressing just before serving.

Per Serving: Calories: 286; Total fat: 26g; Saturated fat: 5g; Cholesterol: 15mg; Sodium: 380mg; Carbohydrates: 18g; Fiber: 6g; Sugar: 7g; Protein: 6g

Broccoli Salad with Sweet Lemon Dressing

With chunks of hearty broccoli, crisp red onion, crunchy sunflower seeds, tangy dried cranberries, and sweet, lemony, yogurt dressing, this salad is sure to be gobbled up by the entire family. It's also an easy and delicious way to check off several MIND diet foods in a single serving.

FOR THE DRESSING

- ½ cup plain yogurt (not Greek)
- 2 tablespoons honey or granulated sugar
- 2 tablespoons mayonnaise
- 2 tablespoons apple cider vinegar
- Zest and juice of 1 medium lemon (about 2 tablespoons)
- ½ teaspoon kosher or sea salt

FOR THE SALAD

- 2 medium heads broccoli, chopped into bite-size pieces (about 5 cups)
- ¼ medium red onion, peeled and finely diced
- ½ cup roasted sunflower seeds
- ½ cup unsweetened, dried cranberries

GLUTEN-FREE
NUT-FREE
VEGETARIAN

Serves: 6

Prep Time: 15 to 20 minutes

Substitution tip
For a vegan salad, use vegan yogurt and mayonnaise and use the granulated sugar rather than the honey for the dressing.

Variation tip
Swap out half of the broccoli for chopped cauliflower.

1. To make the dressing, in a medium bowl, whisk together the yogurt, honey, mayonnaise, vinegar, lemon zest and juice, and salt. Taste and adjust seasoning, if necessary.

2. To make the salad, in a large bowl, toss together the broccoli, onion, sunflower seeds, and dried cranberries. Toss with the dressing and refrigerate at least 30 minutes.

3. The broccoli salad can be prepped in advance and stored in an airtight container for up to 3 days in the refrigerator.

Per Serving: Calories: 139; Total fat: 9g; Saturated fat: 1g; Cholesterol: 3mg; Sodium: 208mg; Carbohydrates: 13g; Fiber: 3g; Sugar: 8g; Protein: 4g

Spinach, Walnut, and Goat Cheese Salad with Raspberry Vinaigrette

The raspberry vinaigrette is truly the star of the show here. It's subtly sweet from both the raspberries and the honey, slightly tangy from the Dijon mustard and red wine vinegar, has undertones of fresh orange, and couldn't be more delicious. It's especially dynamite when paired with the crunchy walnuts, sweet mandarin oranges, and creamy goat cheese on top of a bed of greens.

FOR THE DRESSING
- 1 cup fresh raspberries
- Zest and juice of ½ orange (about ¼ cup)
- ¼ cup extra-virgin olive oil
- 1 tablespoon red wine vinegar
- 1 tablespoon honey or granulated sugar
- 1 teaspoon Dijon mustard

¼ teaspoon kosher or sea salt

FOR THE SALAD
- ½ cup chopped walnuts
- 5 cups fresh baby spinach
- ½ cup mandarin oranges, drained
- ¼ cup crumbled goat cheese

GLUTEN-FREE VEGETARIAN

Serves: 6

Prep Time: 10 to 15 minutes

Substitution tip
Omit the goat cheese for a dairy-free salad. Swap in maple syrup or sugar instead of honey for a vegan salad.

Variation tip
Try a mix of chopped kale, Swiss chard, and mustard greens rather than spinach.

1. To make the dressing, in the bowl of a blender or food processor, combine the raspberries, orange zest and juice, olive oil, vinegar, honey, mustard, and salt. Purée until smooth. Taste and adjust seasoning, if necessary.

2. To make the salad, heat a small sauté pan or skillet over medium-low heat. Add the walnuts to the dry skillet and toast for about 60 seconds, tossing frequently, until lightly browned. Set aside to cool.

3. Build the salads in bowls with spinach, oranges, goat cheese, and toasted walnuts. Drizzle with raspberry dressing.

4. The raspberry dressing can be prepped in advance and stored in a separate airtight container for up to 3 days in the refrigerator. The spinach salad can be prepped in advance and stored in airtight containers for up to 3 days in the refrigerator. Drizzle the salad with dressing just before serving.

Per Serving: Calories: 195; Total fat: 17g; Saturated fat: 3g; Cholesterol: 2mg; Sodium: 94mg; Carbohydrates: 10g; Fiber: 3g; Sugar: 6g; Protein: 4g

Herb and Dijon Potato Salad

We love potato salad in the Midwest. I didn't grow up eating it with an herby vinaigrette-style dressing, but I'm hooked. There is so much flavor from the parsley, oregano, and dill that you truly won't miss the mayonnaise. Plus, it allows the hearty potatoes, hard-boiled eggs, and celery to shine.

FOR THE SALAD

- 2 pounds Yukon Gold potatoes, cubed
- 6 large hard-boiled eggs, quartered
- 4 celery stalks, diced
- ½ cup chopped fresh flat-leaf Italian parsley
- 2 tablespoons chopped fresh oregano
- 2 tablespoons chopped fresh dill

FOR THE DRESSING

- ½ cup extra-virgin olive oil
- 3 tablespoons Dijon mustard
- 2 tablespoons white wine vinegar
- 1 tablespoon honey or granulated sugar
- 1 teaspoon kosher or sea salt
- ½ teaspoon freshly ground black pepper

DAIRY-FREE
GLUTEN-FREE
NUT-FREE
VEGETARIAN

Serves: 8
Prep Time: 10 to 15 minutes
Cook Time: 10 to 15 minutes

Cooking tip

To hard-boil eggs, bring a medium saucepan of water to a boil. Use a slotted spoon to gently place each egg into the pot. Place the lid on the pot and cook for 12 to 13 minutes. Drain the pot and fill with cold water and ice. Let cool for 15 minutes, then crack and peel on a paper towel. Rinse each egg under cold water to remove bits of shell.

Variation tip

Try baby red potatoes instead of Yukon Gold.

1. To make the salad, in a large stock pot, bring a gallon of water to a boil. Add the potatoes and cook for about 10 minutes, until just fork-tender. Drain and gently rinse with cold water.

2. In a large bowl, combine the cooled potatoes, hard-boiled eggs, celery, parsley, oregano, and dill.

3. To make the dressing, in a small bowl whisk together the olive oil, mustard, vinegar, honey, salt, and pepper. Taste and adjust seasoning, if necessary. Fold the dressing into the potato salad. Refrigerate at least 30 minutes before serving.

4. The potato salad can be prepped in advance and stored in an airtight container for up to 3 days in the refrigerator.

Per Serving: Calories: 299; Total fat: 17g; Saturated fat: 3g; Cholesterol: 139mg; Sodium: 295mg; Carbohydrates: 14g; Fiber: 1g; Sugar: 3g; Protein: 5g

Summer Watermelon Gazpacho

Think of this gazpacho as a sweet-and-savory veggie smoothie made creamy with coconut milk and avocado. The watermelon, lime, and mint shine through and the jalapeño gives a little kick. It's refreshing, nourishing, and totally delicious.

- ½ mini seedless watermelon, peeled and cubed (about 4 cups)
- 1 medium English cucumber, chopped (about 2 cups)
- 1 medium avocado, halved, pitted, and peeled
- ½ medium red onion, peeled and quartered
- ½ cup canned, full-fat coconut milk
- ¼ cup fresh mint leaves
- ¼ cup fresh basil leaves
- Zest and juice of 3 medium limes (about 6 tablespoons)
- ½ medium jalapeño, seeded and halved
- 1 tablespoon white wine vinegar
- 2 teaspoons kosher or sea salt
- ½ teaspoon freshly ground black pepper

GLUTEN-FREE
NUT-FREE
VEGAN

Serves: 6
Prep Time: 15 to 20 minutes

Cooking tip
For a spicier soup, use the whole jalapeño and for a less spicy soup, use ¼ of the jalapeño or omit altogether.

Substitution tip
Swap the white wine vinegar for red wine vinegar.

1. In a blender, combine the watermelon, cucumber, avocado, onion, coconut milk, mint, basil, lime zest and juice, jalapeño, vinegar, salt, and pepper and purée until smooth. Taste and adjust seasoning, if necessary. Refrigerate at least 1 hour before serving.

2. The gazpacho can be prepped in advance and stored in an airtight container in the refrigerator for up to 3 days.

Per Serving: Calories: 112; Total fat: 7g; Saturated fat: 3g; Cholesterol: 0mg; Sodium: 380mg; Carbohydrates: 14g; Fiber: 3g; Sugar: 8g; Protein: 2g

Creamy Carrot-Ginger Soup

Carrots often take the back seat in recipes, but this time they're front and center. This creamy colorful soup is puréed with apple, ginger, nutmeg, coconut milk, balsamic vinegar, and maple syrup and is packed with beta carotene and fiber. If you're not in the mood for carrots, try butternut squash, parsnips, or beets as the main ingredient.

- 2 tablespoons avocado oil
- ½ medium yellow onion, peeled and diced
- 8 medium carrots, peeled and sliced (about 5 cups)
- 1 medium apple, diced, skin on (about 1 cup)
- 2-inch piece fresh ginger, peeled and minced

1¼ teaspoons kosher or sea salt

1 teaspoon ground nutmeg

¼ teaspoon freshly ground black pepper

¼ teaspoon ground cayenne pepper

3 cups unsalted vegetable stock

½ cup canned, full-fat coconut milk

3 tablespoons maple syrup

1½ tablespoons balsamic vinegar

GLUTEN-FREE
NUT-FREE
VEGAN

Serves: 6
Prep Time: 15 to 20 minutes
Cook Time: 30 to 35 minutes

Substitution tip
Swap out carrots for 5 cups peeled and cubed butternut squash.

Cooking tip
If you don't have an immersion blender, you can use a regular blender to purée the soup. Let soup cool slightly, then carefully transfer it to a blender. If the soup is steaming, remove the plastic knob on the lid and place a kitchen towel over it as you blend to allow some of the steam to escape.

1. In a stock pot or Dutch oven, heat the oil over medium heat. Add the onion and sauté for 4 to 5 minutes, until softened. Stir in the carrots and apple and sauté for another 2 to 3 minutes. Stir in the ginger, salt, nutmeg, pepper, and cayenne.

2. Add the stock and bring to a simmer for about 15 to 20 minutes, stirring occasionally, until the vegetables are very soft. Use an immersion blender to purée soup until smooth. Stir in the coconut milk, maple syrup, and balsamic vinegar. Taste and adjust seasoning, if necessary.

3. The carrot soup can be prepped in advance and stored in airtight containers in the refrigerator for up to 5 days. Reheat in the microwave on high for 2 to 3 minutes, or until heated through.

Per Serving: Calories: 171; Total fat: 8g; Saturated fat: 3g; Cholesterol: 0mg; Sodium: 496mg; Carbohydrates: 25g; Fiber: 3g; Sugar: 17g; Protein: 1g

Zuppa Toscana

This lightened-up version of Zuppa Toscana *has all the flavor of the original with loads of garlic, turkey sausage, Yukon Gold potatoes, and Italian seasonings, with a little zip from red pepper flakes. It's finished with evaporated milk for a rich creaminess, and will leave your house smelling like heaven.*

- 1 tablespoon extra-virgin olive oil
- ½ medium yellow onion, peeled and diced
- 8 ounces ground turkey Italian sausage
- 4 cups chopped kale or baby spinach leaves
- 8 garlic cloves, peeled and minced
- 4 medium Yukon Gold potatoes, diced (about 4 cups)

1 tablespoon Italian seasoning

1 teaspoon kosher or sea salt

½ teaspoon freshly ground black pepper

¼ teaspoon red pepper flakes

4½ cups unsalted chicken stock

¾ cup evaporated milk

GLUTEN-FREE
NUT-FREE

Serves: 8
Prep Time: 10 to 15 minutes
Cook Time: 20 to 25 minutes

Substitution tip
For a lower-carb version, swap out the potatoes for cauliflower florets.

Cooking tip
To make your own "sausage," mix 1 pound ground turkey or chicken with 2 teaspoons fennel seed, 2 teaspoons onion powder, 1 teaspoon garlic powder, 1 teaspoon dried basil leaves, and 1 teaspoon sweet paprika.

1. In a stock pot or Dutch oven, heat the olive oil over medium heat. Add the onion and sauté for 4 to 5 minutes, until softened. Stir in the Italian sausage and sauté for another 5 to 6 minutes, breaking up the sausage with a wooden spoon as it cooks. Stir in the kale and garlic and cook for another 2 to 3 minutes, until the kale has wilted. Stir in the potatoes, Italian seasoning, salt, pepper, and red pepper flakes.

2. Add the stock and bring to a simmer for 10 to 15 minutes, stirring occasionally, until the potatoes are *al dente*. Stir in the evaporated milk and cook for an additional 3 to 5 minutes. Taste and adjust seasoning, if necessary.

3. The soup can be prepped in advance and stored in airtight containers in the refrigerator for up to 5 days. Reheat in the microwave on high for 2 to 3 minutes, or until heated through.

Per Serving: Calories: 143; Total fat: 5g; Saturated fat: 2g; Cholesterol: 23mg; Sodium: 447mg; Carbohydrates: 19g; Fiber: 2g; Sugar: 3g; Protein: 12g

Lemon Chicken Orzo Soup

You know how they say chicken soup warms the soul? Well, I'm pretty sure they were referring to this chicken soup. It's cozy, comforting, and has loads of shredded chicken, vegetables, pasta, and fresh lemon. This soup makes the perfect cozy meal with a hunk of crusty bread.

- 3 tablespoons extra-virgin olive oil
- 1 pound boneless, skinless chicken breasts
- 3 medium carrots, peeled and sliced
- 1 medium yellow onion, peeled and diced
- 4 cups fresh baby spinach or chopped kale
- 6 garlic cloves, peeled and minced
- 1½ teaspoons poultry seasoning

- 1¾ teaspoons kosher or sea salt
- ½ teaspoon freshly ground black pepper
- 6 cups unsalted chicken stock
- 1 tablespoon unsalted all-natural bouillon (optional)
- Zest and juice of 2 medium lemons (about ¼ cup each)
- 1 cup whole-grain orzo
- 1 bay leaf

DAIRY-FREE
NUT-FREE

Serves: 8
Prep Time: 10 to 15 minutes
Cook Time: 30 to 35 minutes

Cooking tip
You can also dice the raw chicken before adding it to the pot. This allows you to skip the step of removing it from the pot and shredding it.

Substitution tip
If you cannot find whole-grain orzo, use regular orzo or another small, shaped, whole-grain pasta.

1. In a Dutch oven or large stock pot, heat the olive oil over medium heat. Add the chicken and cook for 5 to 6 minutes per side, until lightly browned. Remove the chicken from the pot and set aside.

2. Add the carrots and onion to the pot and sauté for 4 to 5 minutes, or until slightly soft. Stir in the spinach and garlic and sauté for another 2 to 3 minutes, or until the greens are wilted. Stir in the poultry seasoning, salt, and pepper.

3. Put the chicken back in the pot, then add the stock, bouillon (if using), and lemon zest and juice. Bring to a simmer, then add the orzo and bay leaf. Cook for 10 to 15 minutes, or until the orzo is *al dente* and chicken is fully cooked. Remove the bay leaf and discard.

4. Using tongs, transfer the chicken breasts to a cutting board and shred with two forks. Return to the pot. Taste and adjust seasoning, if necessary.

5. The orzo soup can be prepped in advance and stored in airtight containers in the refrigerator for up to 5 days. Reheat in the microwave on high for 2 to 3 minutes, or until heated through.

Per Serving: Calories: 241; Total fat: 7g; Saturated fat: 1g; Cholesterol: 28mg; Sodium: 492mg; Carbohydrates: 27g; Fiber: 3g; Sugar: 4g; Protein: 18g

Chipotle Chicken Chili

I love cozying up with a bowl of chili on a brisk fall day. This version is made smoky from the chipotle chile and fire-roasted tomatoes, and includes a load of colorful vegetables and warm spices. I like to top it with diced avocado for a boost of monounsaturated fats and creamy richness.

- 1 tablespoon extra-virgin olive oil
- 1 medium yellow onion, peeled and diced
- 1 medium bell pepper, diced
- 1 pound ground chicken or turkey
- 3 garlic cloves, peeled and minced
- 4 cups baby spinach leaves or chopped kale

3 tablespoons chili powder

1 tablespoon ground cumin

1½ teaspoons kosher or sea salt

½ teaspoon freshly ground black pepper

½ teaspoon dried oregano leaves (optional)

2 chipotle chiles in adobo sauce, chopped

- 2 (15-ounce) cans no-salt-added, fire-roasted diced tomatoes
- 2 (15-ounce) cans no-salt-added, dark red kidney beans, rinsed and drained

2 cups unsalted chicken stock

½ teaspoon brown or granulated sugar (optional)

- 1 medium avocado, peeled, pitted, and diced

DAIRY-FREE
GLUTEN-FREE
NUT-FREE

Serves: 8
Prep Time: 15 to 20 minutes
Cook Time: 25 to 30 minutes

Substitution tip
For vegan chili, substitute the ground chicken or turkey with a can of no-salt-added black beans.

Variation tip
Try diced boneless skinless chicken breast instead of ground.

1. In a Dutch oven or large stock pot, heat the olive oil over medium heat. Add the onion and bell pepper and sauté for 4 to 5 minutes, until slightly soft. Stir in the chicken and sauté for another 5 to 6 minutes, breaking up the meat with a wooden spoon as it cooks. Stir in the garlic and spinach and cook for another 2 to 3 minutes, until the spinach has wilted. Stir in the chili powder, cumin, salt, pepper, oregano (if using), and chipotle chiles.

2. Add the tomatoes and their juices, kidney beans, and stock. Bring to a simmer for 10 to 15 minutes. Stir in the sugar (if using). Taste and adjust seasoning, if necessary. Serve chili topped with diced avocado.

3. The chicken chili can be prepped in advance and stored in airtight containers in the refrigerator for up to 5 days. Reheat in the microwave on high for 2 to 3 minutes, or until heated through. Top with avocado before serving.

Per Serving: Calories: 266; Total fat: 10g; Saturated fat: 1g; Cholesterol: 11mg; Sodium: 440mg; Carbohydrates: 28g; Fiber: 12g; Sugar: 5g; Protein: 24g

Spicy Smashed Pinto Beans

I never considered making my own refried beans, but now that I have, I'll never go back. There is so much flavor from the jalapeño, garlic, cumin, cilantro, and lime. You can smear these beans on tostadas or top them with salsa and serve them with chips. Either way, I can guarantee they'll be gone in no time.

- 1 tablespoon extra-virgin olive oil
- 1 medium yellow onion, peeled and minced
- ½ medium jalapeño, seeded and minced
- 3 garlic cloves, peeled and minced
- 1 tablespoon chili powder
- 1 teaspoon ground cumin
- ¾ teaspoon kosher or sea salt
- ½ teaspoon freshly ground black pepper
- 2 (15-ounce) cans no-salt-added pinto beans, rinsed and drained
- ½ cup unsalted vegetable stock or water
- ¼ cup chopped fresh cilantro
- Zest and juice of ½ medium lime (about 1 tablespoon each)

GLUTEN-FREE
NUT-FREE
VEGAN

Serves: 8
Prep Time: 10 to 15 minutes
Cook Time: 15 to 20 minutes

Variation tip
Try black beans instead of pinto beans, or one can of each.

Substitution tip
Omit the jalapeño for a milder version.

1. In a large saucepan, heat the olive oil over medium heat. Add the onion and jalapeño and sauté for 4 to 5 minutes, until slightly soft. Stir in the garlic and sauté for another 30 to 60 seconds, until fragrant. Stir in the chili powder, cumin, salt, and pepper.

2. Add the beans and stock. Bring to a low simmer for 10 to 15 minutes. Stir in the cilantro and lime zest and juice. Use a potato masher to mash beans as desired. Taste and adjust seasoning, if necessary.

3. The smashed beans can be prepped in advance and stored in an airtight container in the refrigerator for up to 5 days. Reheat in the microwave on high for 2 to 3 minutes, or until heated through.

Per Serving: Calories: 141; Total fat: 3g; Saturated fat: 0g; Cholesterol: 0mg; Sodium: 170mg; Carbohydrates: 23g; Fiber: 6g; Sugar: 2g; Protein: 7g

Roasted Cauliflower with Lemon-Tahini Sauce

Tahini is a nut butter–like paste made from sesame seeds, often used to make hummus. In this recipe, it's mixed with lemon and garlic and drizzled over roasted cauliflower for the ultimate cozy, plant-based side dish.

FOR THE SAUCE

- ¼ cup tahini (sesame seed paste)
- 3 tablespoons extra-virgin olive oil
- Zest and juice of 2 medium lemons (about ¼ cup each)
- 2 garlic cloves, peeled and minced

¼ teaspoon kosher or sea salt

¼ teaspoon freshly ground black pepper

¼ teaspoon red pepper flakes

FOR THE CAULIFLOWER

- 1 medium cauliflower head, trimmed and cut into florets (about 5 cups)
- 2 tablespoons extra-virgin olive oil

½ teaspoon kosher or sea salt

¼ teaspoon freshly ground black pepper

¼ cup chopped, fresh, flat-leaf Italian parsley

GLUTEN-FREE
NUT-FREE
VEGAN

Serves: 6
Prep Time: 10 to 15 minutes
Cook Time: 15 to 20 minutes

Variation tip
Add a can of rinsed and drained chickpeas for a higher-protein side dish or meal.

Substitution tip
Swap red pepper flakes for sriracha.

1. Preheat the oven to 400°F.

2. To make the sauce, in a bowl, whisk together the tahini, olive oil, lemon zest and juice, garlic, salt, pepper, and red pepper flakes. Taste and adjust seasoning, if necessary. Set aside.

3. To make the cauliflower, on a baking sheet, place the cauliflower and toss with olive oil, salt, and pepper. Roast for 15 to 20 minutes, until the cauliflower is *al dente* and lightly browned on the outside.

4. Toss the roasted cauliflower with the parsley and drizzle with tahini sauce.

5. The roasted cauliflower and tahini sauce can be prepped in advance and stored in an airtight container for up to 4 days in the refrigerator.

Per Serving: Calories: 225; Total fat: 20g; Saturated fat: 3g; Cholesterol: 0mg; Sodium: 106mg; Carbohydrates: 7g; Fiber: 3g; Sugar: 2g; Protein: 6g

Balsamic-Roasted Beets

Who knew something so simple could be so delicious? These beets are tossed in warm, sweet spices and balsamic vinegar, and are roasted until fork-tender. Not only are they scrumptious, beets are loaded with folate, vitamin C, and fiber.

- 8 medium beets, washed
- 2 tablespoons extra-virgin olive oil, divided
- 1 tablespoon balsamic vinegar
- ½ teaspoon ground cinnamon
- ⅛ teaspoon ground cloves
- ½ teaspoon kosher or sea salt
- ½ teaspoon freshly ground black pepper
- 1 tablespoon honey (optional)

DAIRY-FREE
GLUTEN-FREE
NUT-FREE
VEGETARIAN

Serves: 4

Prep Time: 5 to 10 minutes

Cook Time: 60 to 70 minutes

Variation tip
Sprinkle with chopped fresh thyme to serve.

Substitution tip
Try Jerusalem artichokes instead of beets.

1. Preheat the oven to 375°F.

2. Place the beets in a baking dish and rub with 1 tablespoon olive oil. Cover with aluminum foil and roast for 45 to 55 minutes, or until slightly tender.

3. Remove from the oven and let cool slightly. Peel the skins off and discard.

4. In a small bowl, whisk together the remaining 1 tablespoon olive oil, balsamic vinegar, cinnamon, and cloves. Rub the peeled beets with the oil and vinegar mixture and toss with the salt and pepper. Place back in the baking dish, uncovered, and roast an additional 15 minutes, until fork-tender. Drizzle with honey (if using).

5. The roasted beets can be prepped in advance and stored in airtight containers in the refrigerator for up to 5 days. Reheat in the microwave on high for 1½ to 2 minutes, or until heated through.

Per Serving: Calories: 138; Total fat: 7g; Saturated fat: 1g; Cholesterol: 0mg; Sodium: 268mg; Carbohydrates: 18g; Fiber: 5g; Sugar: 13g; Protein: 3g

Apple, Kohlrabi, and Kale Slaw

Kohlrabi is an oft forgotten nonstarchy vegetable with loads of vitamin C. It pairs nicely with sweet apples and hearty kale, and when served next to Barbecue Spice-Roasted Chicken Legs (page 127), it makes for a filling and satisfying meal.

FOR THE DRESSING

- ½ cup plain yogurt (not Greek)

2 tablespoons honey or granulated sugar

2 tablespoons mayonnaise

2 tablespoons white wine vinegar or champagne vinegar

- Zest and juice of 2 medium limes (about 2 tablespoons each)

½ teaspoon kosher or sea salt

FOR THE SLAW

- 2 medium firm apples, cored and shredded
- 1 medium head kohlrabi, peeled and shredded
- ½ bunch kale, stemmed and chopped

½ cup unsweetened, dried cherries

- ½ cup slivered almonds

GLUTEN-FREE
VEGETARIAN

Serves: 6
Prep Time: 10 to 15 minutes

Cooking tip
Use the greens of the kohlrabi plant in soups, stews, casseroles, and breakfast skillets.

Variation tip
Try shredded green or purple cabbage instead of kohlrabi.

1. To make the dressing, in a medium bowl, whisk together the yogurt, honey, mayonnaise, vinegar, lime zest and juice, and salt. Taste and adjust seasoning, if necessary.

2. To make the slaw, in a large bowl, combine the apples, kohlrabi, kale, cherries, and almonds. Toss with the dressing and refrigerate at least 30 minutes.

3. The slaw can be prepped in advance and stored in an airtight container for up to 3 days in the refrigerator.

Per Serving: Calories: 166; Total fat: 9g; Saturated fat: 1g; Cholesterol: 3mg; Sodium: 154mg; Carbohydrates: 20g; Fiber: 6g; Sugar: 14g; Protein: 5g

Kung Pao Brussels Sprouts

Searing Brussels sprouts in a hot skillet provides that caramelized, crunchy exterior we all know and love. This version is elevated when the sprouts are tossed with an Asian-inspired spicy sauce made from Thai chiles. Be sure to finish it off with crunchy peanuts and scallions for a flavor explosion.

**FOR THE
BRUSSELS SPROUTS**

- 2 tablespoons avocado oil
- 1 pound Brussels sprouts, trimmed and sliced in half (about 3 cups)

½ teaspoon kosher or sea salt

¼ teaspoon freshly ground black pepper

FOR THE SAUCE

¼ cup unsalted vegetable stock

2 teaspoons cornstarch

2 tablespoons low-sodium soy sauce

1 tablespoon rice wine vinegar

1 to 2 tablespoons granulated sugar or honey

- 2 garlic cloves, peeled and minced
- 1-inch piece fresh ginger, peeled and minced

2 dried Thai chiles, crushed

- 1 teaspoon sesame oil
- 2 medium scallions, both green and white parts, thinly sliced (optional)
- ¼ cup crushed roasted peanuts (optional)

**DAIRY-FREE
VEGETARIAN**

Serves: 4

Prep Time: 10 to 15 minutes

Cook Time: 10 to 15 minutes

Cooking tip
If you don't have dried Thai chiles, use ½ teaspoon red pepper flakes instead.

Variation tip
Try this recipe with broccoli rather than Brussels sprouts.

1. To make the Brussels sprouts, in a large sauté pan or skillet, heat the oil over medium heat. Add the Brussels sprouts and sauté for 7 to 8 minutes, or until *al dente*, stirring occasionally. Season with salt and pepper.

2. To make the sauce, in a small bowl, whisk together the stock and cornstarch until dissolved. Whisk in the soy sauce, vinegar, sugar, garlic, ginger, chiles, and sesame oil until combined. Pour the sauce into the skillet with the Brussels sprouts and bring to a simmer for 2 to 3 minutes or until thickened, stirring frequently.

3. Serve the Brussels sprouts topped with scallions (if using) and crushed peanuts (if using).

4. The Brussels sprouts can be prepped in advance and stored in airtight containers in the refrigerator for up to 5 days. Reheat in the microwave on high for 1½ to 2 minutes, or until heated through.

Per Serving: Calories: 169; Total fat: 9g; Saturated fat: 1g; Cholesterol: 0mg; Sodium: 414mg; Carbohydrates: 21g; Fiber: 4g; Sugar: 10g; Protein: 5g

Sweet Corn and Zucchini
Gnocchi Skillet, Page 80

CHAPTER SIX
Vegetarian Mains

Heirloom Tomato and Ricotta Toast

One of my favorite ways to serve garden fresh tomatoes is on toast with creamy ricotta, olive oil, and fresh basil. It takes only a few minutes to prepare, but tastes so good alongside a glass of red wine. Plus, it's totally MIND diet–friendly.

½ cup ricotta

▸ Zest of ½ medium lemon (about 1 tablespoon each)

▸ 4 whole-grain bread slices

▸ 1 large ripe heirloom tomato, sliced

¼ cup fresh basil chiffonade

▸ 2 teaspoons extra-virgin olive oil

¼ teaspoon kosher or sea salt

¼ teaspoon freshly ground black pepper

NUT-FREE
VEGETARIAN

Serves: 4

Prep Time: 5 to 10 minutes

Variation tip
Try with mashed avocado instead of ricotta for a dairy-free version.

Substitution tip
Try sliced fresh mozzarella instead of ricotta. Sprinkle the lemon zest on top of the mozzarella when assembling the toasts.

1. In a small bowl, whisk together the ricotta and lemon zest.

2. Toast the slices of bread.

3. Spread the ricotta mixture on each toast. Top each with sliced tomato, then sprinkle with basil, drizzle with olive oil, and sprinkle with salt and pepper. Serve immediately.

4. It is not recommended to make toasts in advance.

Per Serving: Calories: 186; Total fat: 8g; Saturated fat: 3g; Cholesterol: 16mg; Sodium: 97mg; Carbohydrates: 22g; Fiber: 3g; Sugar: 4g; Protein: 8g

Zucchini Noodle Carbonara

While I love a big bowl of pasta now and then, I'm also a fan of swapping in zucchini noodles because we can all use more veggies. Zucchini also tastes so good when sautéed with garlic and with a thick, glossy sauce from the egg yolks. Who knew zucchini could be comfort food?

- 4 medium zucchinis, spiralized
- ¾ teaspoon kosher or sea salt, divided

  ½ cup freshly grated Parmesan cheese, divided
- 3 large egg yolks

  ¾ teaspoon freshly ground black pepper
- 2 tablespoons extra-virgin olive oil
- 3 garlic cloves, peeled and minced

GLUTEN-FREE
NUT-FREE
VEGETARIAN

Serves: 4
Prep Time: 10 to 15 minutes
Cook Time: 10 to 15 minutes

Cooking tip
Salting the spiralized zucchini draws the moisture out, so when you sauté the zucchini, it actually sautés rather than steams.

Variation tip
Try this recipe with butternut squash or sweet potato noodles. For added protein, serve with cooked, chopped, uncured bacon.

1. Lay the zucchini out on a paper towel–lined baking sheet. Sprinkle with ½ teaspoon salt. Let sit for 10 minutes, then pat dry with paper towel.

2. In a small bowl, whisk together ¼ cup of the Parmesan cheese, egg yolks, the remaining ¼ teaspoon salt, and pepper. Set aside.

3. In a large sauté pan or skillet, heat the olive oil over medium heat. Add the spiralized zucchini and sauté for 1 to 2 minutes, until the zucchini is slightly soft. Stir in the garlic and sauté for 30 to 60 seconds, until fragrant. Remove from the heat and stir in the Parmesan-egg mixture, tossing with tongs until the sauce is thickened.

4. Serve zucchini carbonara in bowls topped with remaining ¼ cup Parmesan cheese.

5. The zucchini noodle carbonara can be prepped in advance and stored in airtight containers for up to 2 days in the refrigerator. Reheat in the microwave for 1 to 2 minutes, or until heated through.

Per Serving: Calories: 191; Total fat: 14g; Saturated fat: 4g; Cholesterol: 149mg; Sodium: 462mg; Carbohydrates: 8g; Fiber: 2g; Sugar: 3g; Protein: 8g

Sweet Corn and Zucchini Gnocchi Skillet

With bell pepper, sweet corn, zucchini, and fresh basil, this gnocchi skillet just screams "summer." I like to use produce from my garden to throw together this meal on a warm evening and it feels good knowing it provides a hearty dose of antioxidants, vitamins, and minerals.

- 1 pound whole-grain gnocchi
- 2 tablespoons extra-virgin olive oil
- 4 ears sweet corn, cut from the cob
- 1 medium red bell pepper, diced
- ½ medium yellow onion, peeled and diced
- 2 medium zucchinis, diced
- 4 garlic cloves, peeled and minced
- ½ cup grated Parmesan cheese, divided
- 3 tablespoons half-and-half
- Zest and juice of 1 medium lime (about 2 tablespoons each)
- 1¼ teaspoons kosher or sea salt
- ½ teaspoon freshly ground black pepper
- ½ cup fresh basil chiffonade, divided

NUT-FREE
VEGETARIAN

Serves: 6
Prep Time: 10 to 15 minutes
Cook Time: 15 to 20 minutes

Substitution tip
Try whole-wheat orecchiette or another shaped pasta instead of gnocchi.

Variation tip
For a winter version of this skillet, swap the corn, zucchini, and basil for butternut squash cubes, mushrooms, and thyme.

1. Bring a large stock pot of water to a boil. Add the gnocchi and cook for 4 to 5 minutes, until the gnocchi float to the surface. Drain and set aside.

2. In a large sauté pan or skillet, heat the olive oil over medium heat. Add the sweet corn, bell pepper, and onion and sauté for 4 to 5 minutes, until soft. Stir in the gnocchi, zucchini, and garlic and sauté for 1 to 2 minutes, until the gnocchi is lightly browned. Stir in ¼ cup Parmesan cheese, half-and-half, lime zest and juice, salt, and pepper. Bring to a simmer for 2 to 3 minutes. Stir in a ¼ cup basil.

3. Serve gnocchi skillet in bowls and top with remaining ¼ cup Parmesan cheese and remaining ¼ cup basil.

4. The gnocchi skillet can be prepped in advance and stored in airtight containers for up to 4 days in the refrigerator. Reheat in the microwave for 1 to 2 minutes, or until heated through.

Per Serving: Calories: 285; Total fat: 9g; Saturated fat: 3g; Cholesterol: 10mg; Sodium: 552mg; Carbohydrates: 49g; Fiber: 5g; Sugar: 5g; Protein: 9g

Cajun Red Beans and Rice

It's not difficult to meet the MIND diet recommendations for beans with delicious dishes like this one. Red beans and rice is a traditional southern dish that is loaded with flavor. I use brown rice because it has more B vitamins and fiber than white rice.

- 2 tablespoons extra-virgin olive oil
- 2 medium stalks celery, diced
- 1 medium green bell pepper, diced
- ½ medium yellow onion, peeled and diced
- 4 garlic cloves, peeled and minced

  1 tablespoon Italian seasoning

  2 teaspoons Cajun or creole seasoning

  ¾ teaspoons kosher or sea salt

  ½ teaspoon freshly ground black pepper
- 2 (15-ounce) cans no-salt-added, dark red kidney beans, rinsed and drained

  ½ cup unsalted vegetable stock

  2 bay leaves
- 2 cups cooked brown rice

GLUTEN-FREE
NUT-FREE
VEGAN

Serves: 4
Prep Time: 10 to 15 minutes
Cook Time: 20 to 25 minutes

Cooking tip
Some Cajun and creole seasonings have added salt, so be sure to read the label. If the seasoning does contain added salt, reduce the amount of salt you add to the red beans.

Variation tip
When you're sautéing the vegetables, add a handful of dark leafy greens, such as chopped spinach or kale.

1. In a Dutch oven, heat the olive oil over medium heat. Add the celery, bell pepper, and onion and sauté for 4 to 5 minutes, until soft. Stir in the garlic, Italian seasoning, Cajun seasoning, salt, and pepper.

2. Add the beans, stock, and bay leaves and bring to a simmer for 10 to 15 minutes, stirring occasionally, until slightly thickened. Using tongs, remove the bay leaves and discard. Reduce the heat to low and fold in the brown rice and cook for an additional 10 to 15 minutes, stirring occasionally. Taste and adjust seasoning, if necessary.

3. The red beans and rice can be prepped in advance and stored in airtight containers for up to 4 days in the refrigerator. Reheat in the microwave for 1 to 2 minutes, or until heated through.

Per Serving: Calories: 375; Total fat: 8g; Saturated fat: 1g; Cholesterol: 0mg; Sodium: 420mg; Carbohydrates: 58g; Fiber: 16g; Sugar: 4g; Protein: 13g

Pesto-Roasted Butter Beans

Otherwise known as lima beans, butter beans have a smooth, buttery texture. They make the perfect base for a casserole and, when roasted in pesto, you can't go wrong. I top this dish off with bread crumbs tossed in lemon zest and olive oil for a crispy crunch.

FOR THE PESTO

1 cup fresh basil leaves

▶ 1 cup baby spinach leaves

½ cup grated Parmesan cheese

▶ ½ cup extra-virgin olive oil

▶ ¼ cup pine nuts

▶ 3 to 4 garlic cloves, peeled

½ teaspoon kosher or sea salt

¼ teaspoon freshly ground black pepper

FOR THE BUTTER BEANS

▶ 2 tablespoons extra-virgin olive oil

▶ 1 medium yellow onion, peeled and diced

▶ 4 cups baby spinach leaves or chopped kale

½ teaspoon kosher or sea salt

½ teaspoon freshly ground black pepper

▶ 3 (15-ounce) cans no-salt-added, butter beans, rinsed and drained

FOR THE TOPPING

½ cup panko bread crumbs

2 tablespoons freshly grated Parmesan cheese

▶ Zest of ½ medium lemon (about 1 tablespoon each)

VEGETARIAN

Serves: 8

Prep Time: 10 to 15 minutes

Cook Time: 20 to 25 minutes

Substitution tip
For a gluten-free version, use gluten-free panko bread crumbs

Variation tip
Try with cannellini beans instead of butter beans.

1. Preheat the oven to 375°F.
2. To make the pesto, in the bowl of a food processor, combine the basil, spinach, Parmesan, olive oil, pine nuts, garlic, salt, and pepper and process until a chunky paste forms, scraping the sides of the bowl with a spatula as needed. Taste and adjust seasoning, if necessary.

3. To make the butter beans, in a Dutch oven, heat the olive oil over medium heat. Add the onion and sauté for 4 to 5 minutes, until the onions are soft. Stir in the spinach and cook another 2 to 3 minutes or until spinach is wilted. Stir in the salt and pepper. Stir in the beans and pesto.

4. In a small bowl, stir together the panko bread crumbs, Parmesan, and lemon zest. Sprinkle over the top of the beans. Roast in the oven for 10 to 15 minutes, or until topping is lightly browned.

5. The butter beans can be prepped in advance and stored in airtight containers for up to 4 days in the refrigerator. Reheat in the microwave for 1 to 2 minutes, or until heated through.

Per Serving: Calories: 370; Total fat: 22g; Saturated fat: 4g; Cholesterol: 6mg; Sodium: 307mg; Carbohydrates: 32g; Fiber: 12g; Sugar: 2g; Protein: 13g

Chickpea and Potato Green Curry

I think it's important to have a few "back pocket" recipes that you can throw together on a busy weeknight that also taste delicious. For me, this curry is it. Plus, it contains several handfuls of leafy greens, a few heaping tablespoons of green curry paste, and a small bunch of cilantro—making it truly green.

- 2 tablespoons extra-virgin olive oil
- 1 medium yellow onion, peeled and diced
- 4 cups baby spinach leaves or chopped kale
- 3 garlic cloves, peeled and minced
- 3 tablespoons green curry paste
- 1½ teaspoon kosher or sea salt
- 1 teaspoon garam masala
- ½ teaspoon freshly ground black pepper
- 2 (15-ounce) cans no-salt-added chickpeas, rinsed and drained
- 2 medium Yukon Gold potatoes, diced (about 1½ cups)
- 3 cups unsalted vegetable stock
- ½ cup canned, full-fat coconut milk
- ½ cup chopped fresh cilantro

GLUTEN-FREE
NUT-FREE
VEGAN

Serves: 8
Prep Time: 10 to 15 minutes
Cook Time: 25 to 30 minutes

Substitution tip
To switch things up, try a heartier leafy green like Swiss chard or mustard greens.

Variation tip
Try red or yellow curry paste instead of green.

1. In a Dutch oven, heat the olive oil over medium heat. Add the onion and sauté for 4 to 5 minutes, or until soft. Stir in the spinach and cook another 2 to 3 minutes or until spinach is wilted. Stir in the garlic, curry paste, salt, garam masala, and pepper and sauté for 30 to 60 seconds, until fragrant.

2. Add the chickpeas, potatoes, and stock and bring to a simmer for 15 to 20 minutes, stirring occasionally, until the potatoes are slightly tender. Stir in the coconut milk and cilantro. Taste and adjust seasoning, if necessary.

3. The curry can be prepped in advance and stored in airtight containers for up to 4 days in the refrigerator. Reheat in the microwave for 2 to 3 minutes, or until heated through.

Per Serving: Calories: 301; Total fat: 7g; Saturated fat: 2g; Cholesterol: 0mg; Sodium: 396mg; Carbohydrates: 33g; Fiber: 6g; Sugar: 4g; Protein: 8g

Lemony *Cacio e Pepe* with Arugula

Cacio e pepe *is simply spaghetti with Parmesan or pecorino and lots of black pepper. I've elevated this version to be both MIND diet–friendly with whole-grain pasta and handfuls of fresh arugula to add a bit more flavor. I've included fresh lemon and a few egg yolks for a boost of choline and to add texture to the sauce.*

- 8 ounces whole-grain spaghetti
- 2 tablespoons extra-virgin olive oil
- 1 tablespoon butter
- 1 teaspoon kosher or sea salt
- 1 teaspoon freshly ground black pepper

- Zest and juice of 1 medium lemon (about 2 tablespoons each), divided
- ½ cup freshly grated Parmesan cheese, divided
- 2 large egg yolks
- 3 cups fresh arugula

NUT-FREE
VEGETARIAN

Serves: 6
Prep Time: 10 to 15 minutes
Cook Time: 10 to 15 minutes

Cooking tip
Adding the pasta water back to the pan when you're sautéing helps create a rich, velvety sauce, as does adding egg yolk.

Variation tip
For a boost of protein and fiber, try chickpea or lentil spaghetti.

1. Bring a large stock pot of water to a boil. Cook pasta according to package directions. Reserve ½ cup of the pasta water. Drain.

2. In a large sauté pan or skillet, heat the olive oil and butter over medium heat. Add the salt, pepper, and lemon zest and sauté for 30 to 60 seconds. Add the reserved pasta water and lemon juice and bring to a simmer. Add the cooked spaghetti and ¼ cup Parmesan cheese and toss with tongs until thickened. Remove from the heat and add the egg yolks. Continue to toss with the tongs until the egg yolks are incorporated. Fold in the arugula.

3. Serve pasta in bowls and top with the remaining ¼ cup Parmesan cheese.

4. The *cacio e pepe* can be prepped in advance and stored in airtight containers for up to 4 days in the refrigerator. Reheat in the microwave for 1 to 2 minutes, or until heated through.

Per Serving: Calories: 248; Total fat: 11g; Saturated fat: 4g; Cholesterol: 74mg; Sodium: 350mg; Carbohydrates: 30g; Fiber: 4g; Sugar: 2g; Protein: 8g

Parmesan Polenta with Tomato Puttanesca

Puttanesca is like a zesty marinara. The olives and capers give it a bit of a briny flavor, while the red pepper flakes give it just enough heat. You can make it with canned, crushed tomatoes or try it with fresh tomatoes. Either way, it's the perfect accompaniment to cheesy polenta.

FOR THE TOMATO PUTTANESCA

- 3 tablespoons extra-virgin olive oil
- 4 garlic cloves, peeled and minced
- 2 tablespoons no-salt-added tomato paste

½ teaspoon kosher or sea salt

½ teaspoon freshly ground black pepper

¼ teaspoon red pepper flakes

- 1 (28-ounce) can no-salt-added, crushed tomatoes

- ¼ cup chopped pitted kalamata olives

2 tablespoons capers

1 teaspoon granulated sugar

FOR THE PARMESAN POLENTA

3 cups milk

- ¾ cup yellow polenta

¼ cup freshly grated Parmesan cheese

- 2 tablespoons extra-virgin olive oil

½ teaspoon kosher or sea salt

GLUTEN-FREE
NUT-FREE
VEGETARIAN

Serves: 8
Prep Time: 10 to 15 minutes
Cook Time: 25 to 30 minutes

Cooking tip
If your grocery store doesn't carry a product called polenta, use fine or medium cornmeal.

Variation tip
Use instant polenta for a quicker cooking version.

1. To make the tomato puttanesca, in a Dutch oven, heat the olive oil over medium heat. Add the garlic and tomato paste and sauté for 30 to 60 seconds, until fragrant. Stir in the salt, pepper, and red pepper flakes.

2. Add the tomatoes and bring to a simmer for 10 to 15 minutes, stirring occasionally. Stir in the olives, capers, and sugar. Taste and adjust seasoning, if necessary.

3. Meanwhile, to make the Parmesan polenta, in a medium sauce-pan, bring the milk to a simmer. Whisk in the polenta and continue to stir until thickened, about 5 minutes. Remove from the heat and stir in the Parmesan cheese, olive oil, and salt. Taste and adjust seasoning, if necessary. Serve puttanesca over polenta.

4. The polenta and puttanesca can be prepped in advance and stored in airtight containers for up to 4 days in the refrigerator. Reheat in the microwave for 2 to 3 minutes, or until heated through.

Per Serving: Calories: 210; Total fat: 14g; Saturated fat: 2g; Cholesterol: 3mg; Sodium: 635mg; Carbohydrates: 18g; Fiber: 3g; Sugar: 4g; Protein: 3g

General Tso's Cauliflower

While the cauliflower is the star of the show here, the sticky sauce makes it totally "craveable." Serve this at a party and the entire tray will be gone in minutes—even carnivores will be asking for seconds.

FOR THE CAULIFLOWER

▸ 1 medium cauliflower head, cut into florets (about 5 cups)

▸ 3 tablespoons avocado oil

½ cup cornstarch

1 teaspoon kosher or sea salt

FOR THE SAUCE

½ cup unsalted vegetable stock

2 tablespoons cornstarch

5 tablespoons low-sodium soy sauce

5 tablespoons rice vinegar

¼ cup honey

▸ 2-inch piece fresh ginger, peeled and minced

▸ 3 garlic cloves, peeled and minced

▸ 1 tablespoon no-salt-added tomato paste

▸ 1 tablespoon sesame oil

▸ 3 medium scallions, both green and white parts, thinly sliced

DAIRY-FREE
NUT-FREE
VEGETARIAN

Serves: 6

Prep Time: 10 to 15 minutes

Cook Time: 20 to 25 minutes

Substitution tip
For a gluten-free version, use tamari instead of soy sauce.

Variation tip
For a meat version, try cubed chicken breast instead of cauliflower florets.

1. Preheat the oven to 425°F. Coat a large baking sheet with cooking spray. Set aside.

2. To make the cauliflower, in a large bowl, toss the cauliflower florets and oil together until evenly coated. In a small bowl, whisk together the cornstarch and salt. Pour the mixture over the cauliflower and toss to evenly coat. Place on the prepared baking sheet in a single layer and roast for 15 to 20 minutes, until lightly browned.

3. Meanwhile, to make the sauce, in a large pot, whisk together the stock and cornstarch until dissolved. Whisk in the soy sauce, rice vinegar, honey, ginger, garlic, tomato paste, and sesame oil until combined. Adjust the heat to medium-high and bring to a simmer, whisking constantly, until thickened. Remove from the heat.

4. Add the cauliflower to the pan with the sauce and toss to combine. Transfer to plates and top with scallions. Serve immediately.

5. The General Tso's cauliflower can be prepped in advance and stored in airtight containers for up to 3 days in the refrigerator. Reheat under the broiler on the middle rack for 10 to 15 minutes, or until heated through.

Per Serving: Calories: 166; Total fat: 3g; Saturated fat: 0g; Cholesterol: 0mg; Sodium: 592mg; Carbohydrates: 33g; Fiber: 2g; Sugar: 15g; Protein: 4g

Sweet Potato Falafel

Falafel is traditionally made with fava beans, but is often made with chickpeas. I've elevated the nutrition by adding sweet potato, as it's a great source of beta carotene. I like to serve the falafel in a big bowl with leafy greens, edamame, mango, and a drizzle of the chipotle aioli.

- 1 (15-ounce) can no-salt-added chickpeas, rinsed and drained
- 1 medium onion, peeled and quartered
- ½ cup fresh cilantro
- ½ cup panko bread crumbs
- 2 garlic cloves, peeled
- 1 teaspoon chili powder
- 1 teaspoon ground cumin
- ¾ teaspoon kosher or sea salt
- ½ teaspoon freshly ground black pepper
- 1 cup cooked, mashed sweet potato
- 1 tablespoon extra-virgin olive oil

NUT-FREE
VEGAN

Serves: 4
Prep Time: 10 to 15 minutes
Cook Time: 20 to 25 minutes

Cooking tip
Spraying the falafel with cooking spray prior to baking will help create a crispy browned crust. Serve with chipotle dipping sauce: To make it, whisk together ¼ cup plain yogurt (not Greek), 3 tablespoons mayonnaise, 1 chopped chipotle chile in adobo sauce, and the zest and juice of 1 medium lime.

Variation tip
For a more traditional version, try cooked fava beans instead of the sweet potato.

1. Preheat the oven to 375°F. Fit a wire rack inside a baking sheet and coat with cooking spray. Set aside.

2. In the bowl of a food processor, combine the chickpeas, onion, cilantro, bread crumbs, garlic, chili powder, cumin, salt, and pepper. Process until ingredients are chopped. Add the sweet potato and olive oil and continue to process until a paste is formed, scraping the sides with a spatula as needed.

3. Using a medium cookie scoop, form 2-inch balls and place them on the prepared wire rack, 1 inch apart. Coat the falafel with cooking spray. Bake for 25 to 30 minutes, or until golden brown on the outside.

4. The sweet potato falafel can be prepped in advance and stored in airtight containers for up to 4 days in the refrigerator. Reheat in the microwave for 1 to 2 minutes, or until heated through.

Per Serving (3 falafel): Calories 164; Total fat: 2g; Saturated fat: 0g; Cholesterol: 0mg; Sodium: 286mg; Carbohydrates: 28g; Fiber: 3g; Sugar: 5g; Protein: 8g

Avocado-Pea Pesto Pasta

Avocado, spring peas, and fresh basil make for an amazing sauce to toss with pasta. Serve this hot or cold with cherry tomatoes and fresh mozzarella for a caprese-style salad. Not only does the pasta provide a hearty dose of whole grains, but the avocado provides heart-healthy monounsaturated fats and fiber; the peas are a good source of vitamins A and C; the tomatoes are filled with antioxidants; and the walnuts supply a boost of omega-3 fatty acids.

- 6 ounces whole-grain shaped pasta (penne, ziti, rotini, etc.)
- 1 medium avocado, halved, pitted, and peeled
- 1 cup spring peas
- ¼ cup extra-virgin olive oil
- ¼ cup fresh basil leaves
- ¼ cup fresh flat-leaf Italian parsley
- 2 tablespoons chopped walnuts
- Zest and juice of 1 medium lemon (about 2 tablespoons each)
- 3 garlic cloves, peeled
- ½ teaspoon kosher or sea salt
- ¼ teaspoon freshly ground black pepper
- 1½ cups halved cherry tomatoes

VEGAN

Serves: 8
Prep Time: 10 to 15 minutes
Cook Time: 10 to 15 minutes

Substitution tip
For a gluten-free version, use gluten-free pasta.

Variation tip
Try shelled edamame instead of peas.

1. Bring a large pot of water to a boil. Cook the pasta according to package directions. Drain and rinse with cold water. Transfer to a large bowl.

2. In the bowl of a food processor, combine the avocado, peas, olive oil, basil, parsley, walnuts, lemon zest and juice, garlic, salt, and pepper and process until smooth. Taste and adjust seasoning, if necessary.

3. Add the pesto to the bowl with the pasta and toss to combine. Fold in the cherry tomatoes. Refrigerate at least 30 minutes before serving.

4. The pesto pasta can be prepped in advance and stored in airtight containers for up to 4 days in the refrigerator.

Per Serving: Calories: 375; Total fat: 24g; Saturated fat: 5g; Cholesterol: 22mg; Sodium: 570mg; Carbohydrates: 31g; Fiber: 3g; Sugar: 9g; Protein: 11g

Butternut Squash Ravioli

Butternut squash and ricotta are a match made in ravioli heaven. In this version of ravioli, I use wonton wrappers because it's fast and simple. If that wasn't delicious enough, I finish it off with an olive oil, walnut, and sage sauce that is to die for.

- 1¼ cups cooked, mashed butternut squash
- ½ cup ricotta
- ¼ cup freshly grated Parmesan cheese, divided
- 2 tablespoons maple syrup
- 1 teaspoon kosher or sea salt
- ½ teaspoon freshly ground black pepper
- 36 wonton wrappers
- ¼ cup chopped walnuts
- ¼ cup extra-virgin olive oil
- 2 garlic cloves, peeled and minced
- 3 leaves fresh sage chiffonade

1. Bring a large pot of water to a boil.
2. In a medium bowl, stir together the butternut squash, ricotta, 2 tablespoons Parmesan cheese, maple syrup, salt, and pepper until combined. Taste and adjust seasoning, if necessary.
3. Line up 18 of the wonton wrappers on a cutting board. Dollop a tablespoon of butternut squash filling in the middle of each wrapper. Fill a small bowl with water. Dip your fingers in the water and line the edges of each wonton wrapper with water. Place another wonton wrapper over the butternut squash filling of each and press the edges to seal. Use a fork to score the edges. Repeat with remaining wonton wrappers and filling.
4. Using a slotted spoon, place each ravioli into the boiling water. Cook for 5 to 7 minutes, or until the pasta is *al dente*. Using the same spoon, remove the cooked ravioli and divide them between bowls.

VEGETARIAN

Serves: 6

Prep Time: 20 to 25 minutes

Cook Time: 15 to 20 minutes

Cooking tip

You can make mashed butternut squash a few ways: (1) Cut a fresh butternut squash in half and roast at 400°F until flesh is soft, about an hour. Scoop out the flesh and discard the skin. (2) Thaw a bag of frozen butternut squash, place it in a bowl and mash it with the back of a fork. (3) Buy a can of butternut squash purée.

Variation tip

Swap butternut squash for pumpkin purée.

5. Meanwhile, heat a sauté pan or skillet over medium heat. Place the walnuts in the dry skillet and cook for 30 to 60 seconds, shaking the pan carefully, until the walnuts are lightly toasted. Remove from the pan and set aside. Place the skillet back on medium heat and add the olive oil, then the garlic and sage. Sauté for 30 to 60 seconds, until the garlic is fragrant.

6. Drizzle the ravioli with sage-garlic olive oil and top with toasted walnuts and remaining 2 tablespoons Parmesan cheese.

7. The butternut squash ravioli can be prepped in advance and stored in airtight containers for up to 4 days in the refrigerator. Reheat the ravioli by lightly sautéing on both sides in a hot skillet.

Per Serving (3 ravioli): Calories: 313; Total fat: 16g; Saturated fat: 3g; Cholesterol: 17mg; Sodium: 561mg; Carbohydrates: 34g; Fiber: 3g; Sugar: 6g; Protein: 9g

Crispy Buffalo Tofu Bites

If you're on the fence about tofu, this is the recipe to try. It's coated with a flavorful batter and baked until golden and crisp, then tossed in spicy buffalo sauce. To make it MIND diet–friendly and balanced, serve with a large green salad.

FOR THE TOFU BITES

- 1 pound extra firm tofu

¼ cup milk

- 1 large egg

½ cup all-purpose or whole-wheat flour

1 tablespoon cornstarch

1 teaspoon garlic powder

1 teaspoon onion powder

1 teaspoon smoked paprika

½ teaspoon kosher or sea salt

½ teaspoon freshly ground black pepper

FOR THE BUFFALO SAUCE

- 1 tablespoon avocado oil

1 tablespoon all-purpose or whole-wheat flour

½ cup hot sauce

1 teaspoon garlic powder

½ teaspoon onion powder

2 tablespoons unsalted vegetable stock or water

NUT-FREE
VEGETARIAN

Serves: 6

Prep Time: 15 to 20 minutes

Cook Time: 15 to 20 minutes

Cooking tip

Drying out the tofu before cooking allows it to get crispy if you're pan-frying or roasting it. Serve with a yogurt-based ranch dressing for dipping.

Variation tip

For a meat version, try cubed chicken breast.

1. Preheat the oven to 400°F. Fit a baking sheet with a wire rack and coat with cooking spray. Set aside.

2. To make the tofu bites, on a plate lined with a clean kitchen towel, place the tofu. Place another kitchen towel on top of the tofu and then a heavy pot on top. Let sit for 10 to 15 minutes. Change towels if they become soaked.

3. In a medium bowl, whisk together the milk and egg until combined. Break the dried tofu into 1-inch pieces and place them in the bowl. Toss to coat.

4. In another medium bowl, whisk together the flour, cornstarch, garlic powder, onion powder, smoked paprika, salt, and pepper. Working in batches and using tongs, transfer the tofu pieces to the dry ingredient mixture and toss each to coat. Place on the wire rack, about 1 inch apart. Coat with cooking spray. Bake for 20 to 25 minutes, or until crispy and golden brown. Transfer the tofu bites to a large bowl.

5. Meanwhile, to make the buffalo sauce, in a medium saucepan, heat the oil over medium heat. Whisk in the flour and simmer for 1 to 2 minutes. Slowly whisk in the hot sauce, garlic powder, and onion powder. Whisk in the vegetable stock. Bring to a simmer and cook for 5 to 6 minutes, until thickened, whisking constantly. Place the tofu bites in a large bowl, pour buffalo sauce over the bites, and toss or stir to coat. Serve immediately.

6. The buffalo tofu bites can be stored in airtight containers for up to 3 days in the refrigerator. Reheat under the broiler on the middle rack for 10 to 15 minutes, or until heated through.

Per Serving: Calories: 157; Total fat: 7g; Saturated fat: 1g; Cholesterol: 31mg; Sodium: 404mg; Carbohydrates: 17g; Fiber: 2g; Sugar: 1g; Protein: 10g

Maple-Soy-Glazed Tofu Bowls

I love when tofu has a super-crispy browned exterior and is tossed in a sweet and spicy glaze, just like this. When I'm building the bowls to go with it, I grab a variety of colorful vegetables like edamame, bok choy, carrots, radishes, and avocado. If you're feeling sassy, drizzle it with a little sriracha mayo.

FOR THE MAPLE-SOY TOFU

▶ 1 pound extra-firm tofu

¼ cup low-sodium soy sauce

1 tablespoon cornstarch

¼ cup maple syrup

1 teaspoon sriracha (optional)

▶ 2 tablespoons avocado oil

▶ 4 garlic cloves, peeled and minced

▶ 1-inch piece fresh ginger, peeled and minced

FOR THE BOWLS

▶ 2 cups cooked brown rice or quinoa

▶ 2 cups cooked shelled edamame

▶ 1½ cups peeled and shredded carrots

½ cup chopped fresh cilantro

▶ ½ cup chopped peanuts (optional)

▶ 2 medium limes, cut into wedges (optional)

VEGAN

Serves: 6
Prep Time: 10 to 15 minutes
Cook Time: 10 to 15 minutes

Substitution tip
Try honey instead of maple syrup.

Variation tip
Try cooked farro, wheat berries, or kamut instead of brown rice or quinoa. For a seafood version, try with cubed fresh salmon instead of tofu.

1. To make the maple-soy tofu, on a plate lined with a clean kitchen towel, place the tofu. Place another kitchen towel on top of the tofu and then a heavy pot on top. Let sit for 10 to 15 minutes. Change towels if they become soaked. Chop the tofu into 1-inch cubes.

2. In a small bowl, whisk together the soy sauce and cornstarch until dissolved. Whisk in the maple syrup and sriracha (if using). Set aside.

3. In a large sauté pan or skillet, heat the oil over medium-high heat. Add the tofu and sauté for 2 to 3 minutes on each side, until browned and crisp. Stir in the garlic and ginger and sauté for 30 to 60 seconds, until fragrant. Pour the maple-soy mixture into the skillet and bring to a simmer for 1 to 2 minutes, stirring constantly, until thickened. Remove the skillet from the heat.

4. To make the bowls, divide the rice, maple-soy tofu, edamame, carrots, and cilantro between bowls. Top with peanuts (if using), drizzle with the maple-soy sauce, and serve with lime wedges (if using).

5. The maple-soy tofu can be prepped in advance and stored in airtight containers for up to 3 days in the refrigerator. Reheat in the microwave for 1 to 2 minutes, or until heated through. The bowl toppings can be prepped in advance and stored in an airtight container for up to 3 days in the refrigerator. Top bowls with reheated tofu just before serving.

Per Serving: Calories: 364; Total fat: 12g; Saturated fat: 1g; Cholesterol: 0mg; Sodium: 633mg; Carbohydrates: 44g; Fiber: 8g; Sugar: 16g; Protein: 18g

Lentil and Mushroom Bolognese

Both the mushrooms and lentils give this vegetarian Bolognese a meaty texture that goes well with the Italian herbs and red wine. Serve it over pasta with freshly grated Parmesan for the ultimate bowl of comfort.

- ▸ 2 tablespoons extra-virgin olive oil
- ▸ 1 pound mushrooms, diced
- ▸ 2 medium carrots, peeled and diced
- ▸ 1 medium yellow onion, peeled and diced
- ▸ 4 garlic cloves, peeled and minced
-   1½ tablespoons Italian seasoning
-   1½ teaspoons kosher or sea salt
-   ½ teaspoon freshly ground black pepper

- ▸ 1 cup dried red or green lentils
- ▸ ½ cup dry red wine
- ▸ 1 (32-ounce) can no-salt-added, crushed tomatoes
-   3 cups unsalted vegetable stock
-   ½ cup chopped fresh basil (optional)
- ▸ 8 ounces whole-grain spaghetti or linguine (optional)
-   ¼ cup freshly grated Parmesan cheese

**NUT-FREE
VEGETARIAN**

Serves: 8
Prep Time: 10 to 15 minutes
Cook Time: 35 to 40 minutes

Substitution tip
Use nutritional yeast instead of Parmesan cheese to make this dish vegan.

Variation tip
For a meat version, swap out lentils for 8 ounces ground turkey or chicken. Reduce the stock to 1 cup.

1. In a Dutch oven or stock pot, heat the olive oil over medium heat. Add the mushrooms, carrots, and onion and sauté for 6 to 7 minutes, or until the vegetables are soft. Stir in the garlic, Italian seasoning, salt, and pepper and sauté for 30 to 60 seconds, or until the garlic is fragrant. Stir in the lentils. Add the red wine and stir until almost evaporated, turning up the heat if necessary.

2. Add the crushed tomatoes, stock, and basil (if using). Bring to a simmer and cook for 25 to 30 minutes, or until the lentils are *al dente* and the liquid is mostly absorbed, stirring frequently. Run an immersion blender through the sauce for a few seconds to thicken it. Taste and adjust seasoning, if necessary.

3. Bring a large stock pot of water to a boil. Cook pasta (if using) according to package directions. Drain and serve the sauce over the pasta. Top with Parmesan cheese.

4. The Bolognese can be prepped in advance and stored in airtight containers for up to 5 days in the refrigerator. Reheat in the microwave for 1 to 2 minutes, or until heated through.

Per Serving: Calories: 311; Total fat: 6g; Saturated fat: 1g; Cholesterol: 3mg; Sodium: 411mg; Carbohydrates: 45g; Fiber: 10g; Sugar: 15g; Protein: 23g

Grilled Chimichurri Scallops, Page 115

CHAPTER SEVEN
Seafood Mains

Crispy Whitefish with *Arrabiata*

The word arrabiata *means "angry" in Italian because of the red pepper flakes that add quite a bit of heat to this sauce. Don't let that turn you away, though. It's a deliciously rich, tomatoey sauce that pairs perfectly with crispy baked whitefish and freshly shaved Parmesan cheese.*

FOR THE *ARRABIATA*

- 3 tablespoons extra-virgin olive oil
- 4 garlic cloves, peeled and minced
- 2 tablespoons no-salt-added tomato paste

¾ teaspoon red pepper flakes

½ teaspoon kosher or sea salt

½ teaspoon freshly ground black pepper

- 1 (28-ounce) can no-salt-added crushed tomatoes

1 teaspoon granulated sugar

FOR THE CRISPY WHITEFISH

¾ cup all-purpose or whole wheat flour

- 2 large eggs, beaten

2 tablespoons Dijon mustard

1¼ cups panko bread crumbs

1 teaspoon kosher or sea salt, divided

¾ teaspoon freshly ground black pepper, divided

- 1½ pounds whitefish fillets, skin removed

¼ cup freshly grated Parmesan cheese

NUT-FREE

Serves: 6

Prep Time: 10 to 15 minutes

Cook Time: 15 to 20 minutes

Substitution tip
For a gluten-free version, swap the all-purpose flour for gluten-free all-purpose flour.

Substitution tip
Make it dairy-free by omitting the cheese.

1. Preheat the oven to 400°F. Place a wire rack inside a baking sheet and coat with cooking spray.

2. To make the *arrabiata*, in a Dutch oven, heat the olive oil over medium heat. Add the garlic and tomato paste and sauté for 30 to 60 seconds, until fragrant. Stir in the red pepper flakes, salt, and pepper.

3. Add the tomatoes and bring to a simmer for 10 to 15 minutes, stirring occasionally. Stir in the sugar. Taste and adjust seasoning, if necessary.

4. To make the crispy whitefish, set up three bowls: one with flour, one with beaten egg and mustard, and one with bread crumbs. Divide the salt and pepper between the bowls and stir each to combine.

5. Working one at a time, dip the fish fillets into flour, then egg, then the bread crumbs and place on the prepared wire rack. Coat each with cooking spray. Bake for 10 to 15 minutes, until the fish is firm.

6. Transfer to a warmed serving dish and top the crispy fish fillets with *arrabiata* sauce and Parmesan cheese. Serve immediately.

7. The *arrabiata* sauce and crispy fish can be prepped in advance and stored in separate airtight containers for up to 4 days in the refrigerator. Reheat sauce in the microwave for 2 to 3 minutes or until heated through. Reheat the fish by lightly sautéing in a hot skillet on both sides. Spoon *arrabiata* sauce over crispy fish just before serving.

Per Serving: Calories: 368; Total fat: 11g; Saturated fat: 2g; Cholesterol: 114mg; Sodium: 642mg; Carbohydrates: 37g; Fiber: 5g; Sugar: 7g; Protein: 29g

Spicy Fish Taco Bowls with Mango Salsa

This fish taco bowl reminds me of a version I had at a Cuban restaurant in Key West. The chili-dusted fish, brightly colored, crunchy vegetables, and sweet and tangy mango salsa make for bold and exciting bowls that are packed with MIND-friendly ingredients. Plus, they're quick and easy to make.

FOR THE MANGO SALSA

- 2 medium mangos, peeled, pitted, and diced

  ½ cup chopped fresh cilantro

- Zest and juice of 2 medium limes (about 1/4 cup each)

FOR THE TACO BOWLS

- 2 cups cooked brown rice or quinoa

- 1 medium English cucumber, diced

- 1 cup shredded red cabbage

- 2 medium avocados, peeled, pitted, and diced

FOR THE SPICY FISH

- 1 tablespoon extra-virgin olive oil

- 1½ pounds whitefish, skins removed

  1 tablespoon chili powder

  ½ teaspoon kosher or sea salt

  ½ teaspoon freshly ground black pepper

- 2 medium limes, cut into wedges

DAIRY-FREE
GLUTEN-FREE
NUT-FREE

Serves: 6

Prep Time: 10 to 15 minutes

Cook Time: 10 to 15 minutes

Substitution tip
Try pineapple in the salsa instead of mango.

Cooking tip
If you prefer to bake the fish, rub the fish fillets with olive oil and dust with chili powder, salt, and pepper. Bake at 400°F for 8 to 10 minutes.

1. To make the mango salsa, in a medium bowl, stir together the mango, cilantro, and lime zest and juice until combined. Set aside.

2. To make the taco bowls, distribute the cooked rice, cucumber, cabbage, and avocado between bowls. Set aside.

3. To make the spicy fish, in a large nonstick sauté pan or skillet, heat the olive oil over medium heat. Dust the fish with chili powder, salt, and pepper. Once hot, add the fish to the skillet and sauté for 2 to 3 minutes per side, or until the fish flakes easily with a fork.

4. Distribute cooked fish between the bowls and top each with the mango salsa. Serve immediately with lime wedges.

5. The mango salsa and bowl toppings can be prepped in advance and stored in airtight containers in the refrigerator for up to 4 days. The spicy fish can be prepped in advance and stored in airtight containers for up to 3 days in the refrigerator. Reheat in the microwave for 1 to 2 minutes, or until heated through. Add the fish just before serving.

Per Serving: Calories: 359; Total fat: 12g; Saturated fat: 2g; Cholesterol: 49mg; Sodium: 302mg; Carbohydrates: 41g; Fiber: 9g; Sugar: 18g; Protein: 26g

Pan-Roasted Whitefish with Olive Tapenade

A tapenade is simply a French name for finely chopped olives and olive oil that is served as a condiment. In this instance, we're serving up a kalamata and green olive tapenade on simple, pan-roasted whitefish. This dish is a great source of monounsaturated and omega-3 fats, both important for brain health.

FOR THE OLIVE TAPENADE

- ▸ ½ cup pitted kalamata olives
- ▸ ½ cup pitted green olives
  ½ cup fresh flat-leaf parsley
- ▸ ¼ cup extra-virgin olive oil
- ▸ 2 garlic cloves, peeled
  1 teaspoon dried oregano leaves
  ¼ teaspoon freshly ground black pepper

FOR THE PAN-ROASTED WHITEFISH

- ▸ 2 tablespoons extra-virgin olive oil
- ▸ 1½ pounds whitefish fillets, skins removed
  ¼ teaspoon kosher or sea salt
  ¼ teaspoon freshly ground black pepper

DAIRY-FREE
GLUTEN-FREE
NUT-FREE

Serves: 6
Prep Time: 10 to 15 minutes
Cook Time: 10 to 15 minutes

Cooking tip
Try different types of white-fish, such as cod, haddock, halibut, flounder, mahi mahi, or tilapia.

Variation tip
Try 1 tablespoon chopped fresh oregano instead of dried oregano.

1. To make the olive tapenade, in the bowl of a food processor, combine the olives, parsley, olive oil, garlic, oregano, and pepper. Pulse until a pesto-like consistency is reached, scraping the sides of the bowl with a spatula as needed. Set aside.

2. To make the pan-roasted whitefish, in a large nonstick sauté pan or skillet, heat the olive oil over medium-high heat. Season the fish fillets with salt and pepper. Sauté the fish for 2 to 3 minutes per side, or until the fish flakes easily with a fork. Top the fish with olive tapenade. Serve immediately.

3. The olive tapenade can be prepped in advance and stored in airtight containers for up to 7 days in the refrigerator. The pan-roasted fish can be prepped in advance and stored in airtight containers for up to 3 days. Reheat the fish by lightly sautéing in a hot skillet on both sides. Spoon the tapenade over the fish just before serving.

Per Serving: Calories: 290; Total fat: 19g; Saturated fat: 2g; Cholesterol: 66mg; Sodium: 480mg; Carbohydrates: 37g; Fiber: 1g; Sugar: 0g; Protein: 28g

Blackened Catfish with *Pico de Gallo*

Salsas and pico de gallo *are packed with MIND-healthy vegetables and fruits, making them the perfect topping for fish. I like to pair these fresh ingredients with bold spices like those found in blackened and Old Bay seasoning. However, these spice mixtures are often loaded with salt, so it's best to make your own.*

FOR THE *PICO DE GALLO*

- ▶ 4 small ripe tomatoes, stemmed and diced
- ▶ ½ medium white onion, peeled and minced
  ½ cup chopped fresh cilantro
- ▶ Zest and juice of 2 medium limes (about ¼ cup each)
- ▶ ½ medium jalapeño, seeded and minced
  ½ teaspoon kosher or sea salt

¼ teaspoon freshly ground black pepper

FOR THE BLACKENED CATFISH

- ▶ 2 tablespoons extra-virgin olive oil
- ▶ 1½ pounds catfish fillets, skins removed
  1 tablespoon blackened or Old Bay seasoning
  ¼ teaspoon kosher or sea salt

DAIRY-FREE
GLUTEN-FREE
NUT-FREE

Serves: 4
Prep Time: 10 to 15 minutes
Cook Time: 10 to 15 minutes

Cooking tip
To make your own salt-free blackened or Old Bay seasoning, combine 3 tablespoons smoked paprika, 2 teaspoons onion powder, 1 teaspoon garlic powder, 1 teaspoon ground black pepper, 1 teaspoon dried thyme, 1 teaspoon dried oregano, and ½ teaspoon cayenne pepper. Store in an airtight container in the pantry up to 2 months.

Variation tip
Try this recipe with cod, haddock, or halibut.

1. To make the *pico de gallo*, in a medium bowl, mix the tomatoes, onion, cilantro, lime zest and juice, jalapeño, salt, and pepper until combined. Taste and adjust seasoning, if necessary. Set aside.

2. In a large nonstick sauté pan or skillet, heat the olive oil over medium-high heat. Season the catfish fillets with blackened seasoning and salt. Sauté the fish in the oil for 2 to 3 minutes per side, until the fish flakes easily with a fork. Top with *pico de gallo* and serve immediately.

3. The *pico de gallo* can be prepped in advance and stored in airtight containers for up to 3 days in the refrigerator. The blackened catfish can be prepped in advance and stored in airtight containers for up to 3 days. Reheat the fish by lightly sautéing in a hot skillet on both sides. Spoon the *pico de gallo* over the fish just before serving.

Per Serving: Calories: 352; Total fat: 19g; Saturated fat: 4g; Cholesterol: 114mg; Sodium: 437mg; Carbohydrates: 10g; Fiber: 2g; Sugar: 5g; Protein: 33g

Firecracker-Glazed Salmon Nuggets

Salmon is perhaps the most well-known fatty fish that contains a hefty dose of omega-3 fatty acids. Many people are intimidated about cooking fatty fish like salmon, but once you get a little practice, it's quick and simple. My best tip for cooking fish perfectly every time is to use the "fork method." Use the back of a fork to gently press down on the fish fillet; if it springs back, it's not quite done; if it starts to flake, it's ready to eat!

¼ cup buffalo sauce

3 tablespoons dark brown sugar

1 tablespoon apple cider vinegar

1½ teaspoons honey

1 teaspoon cornstarch

¼ teaspoon onion powder

¼ teaspoon garlic powder

¼ teaspoon freshly ground black pepper

▸ 2 tablespoons avocado oil

▸ 1½ pounds salmon, skin removed, cubed

DAIRY-FREE
GLUTEN-FREE
NUT-FREE

Serves: 6

Prep Time: 5 to 10 minutes

Cook Time: 10 to 15 minutes

Substitution tip
If you don't like salmon, try this recipe with whitefish instead.

Variation tip
Serve salmon nuggets in bibb or Boston lettuce leaves with *Pico de Gallo* (page 107) or Mango Salsa (page 104).

1. In a medium bowl, whisk together the buffalo sauce, brown sugar, vinegar, honey, cornstarch, onion powder, garlic powder, and pepper, plus 1½ teaspoons water, until smooth. Set aside.

2. In a large nonstick sauté pan or skillet, heat the oil over medium-high heat. Sauté the salmon for 30 to 60 seconds on each side. Pour the sauce mixture into the skillet and bring to a simmer for 1 to 2 minutes, or until sauce is thickened and the salmon nuggets flake easily with a fork. Serve immediately.

3. The salmon nuggets can be prepped in advance and stored in airtight containers for up to 3 days. Reheat the fish by lightly sautéing in a hot skillet on all sides.

Per Serving: Calories: 140; Total fat: 2g; Saturated fat: 1g; Cholesterol: 45mg; Sodium: 460mg; Carbohydrates: 8g; Fiber: 0g; Sugar: 7g; Protein: 21g

Coconut-Lime Poached Salmon

In this dish, salmon takes a bath with coconut milk, lime juice, fish sauce, ginger, and sriracha and is served with seared baby bok choy, a green leafy vegetable often used in Asian cooking. Be sure to grab a can of coconut milk rather than the jug of coconut milk often found in the dairy alternatives section of the grocery store.

- 1 tablespoon avocado oil
- 4 baby bok choy, sliced in half lengthwise
- 1½ cups unsalted vegetable stock
- ½ cup full-fat, canned coconut milk
- Zest and juice of 2 medium limes (about ¼ cup each)
- 1-inch piece fresh ginger, peeled and minced

- 2 teaspoons dark brown sugar
- 1 teaspoon fish sauce
- 1 teaspoon sriracha
- ½ teaspoon kosher or sea salt
- ½ teaspoon freshly ground black pepper
- 1½ pounds salmon fillets, skins removed
- ¼ cup chopped fresh cilantro

DAIRY-FREE
NUT-FREE

Serves: 4
Prep Time: 10 to 15 minutes
Cook Time: 15 to 20 minutes

Cooking tip
Poaching is a moist-heat cooking method in which food is slow cooked in a liquid that is between 160 and 180°F.

Variation tip
Try with 4 cups of fresh baby spinach, chopped kale, or Swiss chard instead of bok choy.

1. In a shallow Dutch oven or stovetop casserole dish, heat the oil over medium heat. Add the bok choy and sear for 1 to 2 minutes per side, until lightly browned. Using tongs, remove the bok choy from the skillet. Set aside.

2. In the same pot, on medium heat, add the stock, coconut milk, lime zest and juice, ginger, brown sugar, fish sauce, sriracha, salt, and pepper and whisk to combine. Bring to a low simmer. Add the salmon and bok choy and simmer for 8 to 10 minutes, or until the salmon flakes easily with a fork and the boy choy is slightly tender. Taste the poaching liquid and adjust seasoning, if necessary.

3. Serve the fish in bowls, spooning the poaching liquid over the fillets, and top with cilantro.

4. The poached salmon can be prepped in advance and stored in airtight containers for up to 3 days. Reheat the fish in the microwave for 1 to 2 minutes, or until heated through.

Per Serving: Calories: 331; Total fat: 16g; Saturated fat: 6g; Cholesterol: 78mg; Sodium: 523mg; Carbohydrates: 9g; Fiber: 1g; Sugar: 5g; Protein: 37g

Tuna Salad–Stuffed Avocados

If you're not in the mood to cook, this recipe is for you! This simple tuna salad is packed with brain-healthy vegetables and a creamy yogurt dressing. It's stuffed inside avocado halves and topped with scallions to make the ultimate no-cook desk lunch.

- 2 (4-ounce cans) albacore tuna, drained
- 2 medium stalks celery, diced
- ½ medium red onion, peeled and minced
- 3 tablespoons plain Greek yogurt
- 2 tablespoons mayonnaise
- 1 tablespoon Dijon mustard
- Zest and juice of ½ medium lemon (about 1 tablespoon each)

- ½ medium jalapeño, seeded and minced
- ½ teaspoon kosher or sea salt
- ¼ teaspoon freshly ground black pepper
- 2 medium scallions, both white and green parts, thinly sliced, divided
- 3 medium avocados, halved and pitted

GLUTEN-FREE
NUT-FREE

Serves: 6

Prep Time: 10 to 15 minutes

Cooking tip
Adding a little bit of mayonnaise to a yogurt sauce helps cut down on the tanginess of the yogurt and provides a creamy, rich texture. You don't need much and using just a little can easily fit into the MIND diet. If using canned tuna, you can use water- or olive oil-packed tuna. Both are MIND diet-friendly, and the olive oil-packed tuna contains more heart-healthy fats.

Variation tip
Serve tuna salad on whole-grain bread instead of inside avocado halves. Try tuna from the pouch instead of canned.

1. In a medium bowl, stir together the tuna, celery, red onion, Greek yogurt, mayonnaise, mustard, lemon zest and juice, jalapeño, salt, and pepper until combined. Fold in half of the scallions. Taste and adjust seasoning, if necessary.

2. Spoon the tuna salad into the avocado wells. Top with the remaining scallions. Serve immediately.

3. The tuna salad can be prepped in advance and stored in airtight containers in the refrigerator for up to 3 days. Halve and pit avocados just before stuffing.

Per Serving: Calories: 204; Total fat: 15g; Saturated fat: 2g; Cholesterol: 15mg; Sodium: 278mg; Carbohydrates: 9g; Fiber: 6g; Sugar: 2g; Protein: 11g

Sesame-Crusted *Ahi* Tuna with Ponzu Sauce

I couldn't write a brain health book without sharing a recipe for sesame seed–crusted ahi tuna. In additional to being a great source of vitamin E and fiber, sesame seeds also contain lignans and phytosterols that may have cholesterol-lowering effects. Ahi tuna provides a dose of B vitamins and is a lean source of protein, making this a winning combo.

FOR THE PONZU SAUCE

¼ cup low-sodium soy sauce

▸ Zest and juice of 1 medium orange (2 tablespoons each)

▸ Zest and juice of 1 medium lime (about 1 tablespoon each)

1 tablespoon mirin (Japanese sweet rice wine)

⅛ teaspoon red pepper flakes

FOR THE *AHI* TUNA

▸ 2 tablespoons avocado oil

▸ 1 pound *ahi* tuna steaks

¼ teaspoon kosher or sea salt

¼ teaspoon freshly ground black pepper

▸ ¼ cup black and/or white sesame seeds

DAIRY-FREE
NUT-FREE

Serves: 4
Prep Time: 10 to 15 minutes
Cook Time: 10 to 15 minutes

Substitution tip
If you can't find mirin, use 1 tablespoon dry white wine plus 1 teaspoon granulated sugar.

Cooking tip
Choose *ahi* from a reputable seafood market. Consuming undercooked or raw fish may be harmful to health.

1. To make the ponzu sauce, in a medium bowl, whisk together the soy sauce, orange zest and juice, lime zest and juice, mirin, and red pepper flakes. Set aside.

2. To make the *ahi* tuna, in a large sauté pan or skillet, heat the oil over medium heat. Season the tuna steaks with salt and pepper. Place the sesame seeds in a shallow dish. Press all sides of each tuna steak into the sesame seeds. Sear tuna steaks in the oil for 1 to 2 minutes per side and for 1 to 2 minutes on each edge, until all sides are browned and crisp. Serve immediately with ponzu sauce for dipping.

3. The ponzu sauce can be made in advance and stored in an airtight container in the refrigerator for up to 7 days. It is not recommended to cook the tuna in advance. Prepare the tuna just before serving.

Per Serving: Calories: 281; Total fat: 13g; Saturated fat: 2g; Cholesterol: 40mg; Sodium: 610mg; Carbohydrates: 9g; Fiber: 2g; Sugar: 4g; Protein: 33g

Mediterranean Trout *en Papillote*

Cooking fish en papillote *means it's being steamed inside a parchment paper pouch, resulting in a tender and flavorful product. This version has a combination of fennel, lemon, herbs, tomatoes, and olives, but any vegetable-and-herb blend would work.*

- 1 cup baby spinach leaves or chopped kale
- 1½ pounds trout, skins removed
- 1 tablespoon extra-virgin olive oil

  ½ teaspoon kosher or sea salt

  ½ teaspoon freshly ground black pepper

- ½ fennel bulb, thinly sliced
- 1 medium lemon, thinly sliced

  ½ cup fresh dill, parsley, tarragon, and/or chives

- 1 pint cherry tomatoes, halved
- ½ cup pitted kalamata olives

DAIRY-FREE
GLUTEN-FREE
NUT-FREE

Serves: 6
Prep Time: 15 to 20 minutes
Cook Time: 15 to 20 minutes

Substitution tip
Try this with shrimp, salmon, or scallops.

Cooking tip
Use the fennel fronds as a garnish when serving.

1. Preheat the oven to 400°F. Cut two pieces of parchment paper large enough to fold over the fish, with 10 to 15 extra inches for folding. Place the parchment papers on two baking sheets.

2. Place half of the spinach in the center of each piece of parchment paper and the fish fillets on top. Drizzle the olive oil over the fish and sprinkle with salt and pepper. Arrange the fennel, lemon slices, and dill on top of the fish fillets. Arrange the cherry tomatoes and olives tightly around the fish.

3. Fold the parchment in half over the fish, then fold and pinch along the edges to seal. Bake for 15 to 20 minutes. To test for doneness, stick an instant-read thermometer through the parchment into the thickest part of the fish; it's done when it reaches 145 degrees. Remove the packets from the oven and let cool for 2 to 3 minutes. Carefully open the pouches and serve immediately.

4. The trout can be prepped in advance and stored in airtight containers for up to 3 days. Reheat the fish by lightly sautéing in a hot sauté pan or skillet on both sides.

Per Serving: Calories: 268; Total fat: 13g; Saturated fat: 2g; Cholesterol: 67mg; Sodium: 512mg; Carbohydrates: 12g; Fiber: 3g; Sugar: 2g; Protein: 26g

Sheet-Pan Shrimp Boil

I've transformed the shrimp boil into a super-tasty sheet-pan meal. Baby potatoes, sweet corn, and shrimp are doused in olive oil, Old Bay seasoning, garlic, lemon, and parsley and are roasted until caramelized. Serve with some green veggies to make a complete meal.

- 1 pound baby red or Yukon Gold potatoes, halved
- 3 ears sweet corn, cleaned and cut into 3-inch pieces
- 2 pounds large shrimp, peeled and deveined
- 3 tablespoons extra-virgin olive oil, divided
- 1 tablespoon Old Bay or blackened seasoning
- ½ teaspoon kosher or sea salt
- 3 garlic cloves, peeled and minced
- ¼ cup chopped fresh flat-leaf Italian parsley
- 2 medium lemons, cut into wedges

DAIRY-FREE
GLUTEN-FREE
NUT-FREE

Serves: 4
Prep Time: 15 to 20 minutes
Cook Time: 20 to 25 minutes

Cooking tip
To make your own salt-free Old Bay or blackened seasoning, combine 3 tablespoons smoked paprika, 2 teaspoons onion powder, 1 teaspoon garlic powder, 1 teaspoon ground black pepper, 1 teaspoon dried thyme, 1 teaspoon dried oregano, and ½ teaspoon cayenne pepper. Store in an airtight container in the pantry for up to 2 months.

Variation tip
Try this recipe with scallops.

1. Preheat the oven to 400°F. Coat a baking sheet with cooking spray.

2. Bring a large pot of water to a boil. Add the potatoes and cook for 5 minutes. Add the corn to the pot and continue to cook for 5 more minutes. Drain the potatoes and corn and transfer to the prepared baking sheet.

3. Add the shrimp to the baking sheet. Drizzle with 2 tablespoons of olive oil and sprinkle with the Old Bay seasoning and salt and toss the potatoes, corn, and shrimp to coat. Roast for 8 to 10 minutes.

4. In a small bowl, whisk together the remaining 1 tablespoon olive oil and garlic. Add the olive oil and garlic mixture to the baking sheet and stir the potatoes, corn, and shrimp to coat. Roast another 2 to 3 minutes, or until the shrimp is slightly curled and the potatoes and corn are lightly browned. Toss with chopped parsley. Serve immediately with lemon wedges.

5. The shrimp boil can be prepped in advance and stored in airtight containers for up to 3 days. Reheat by lightly sautéing the mixture in a hot sauté pan or skillet on both sides.

Per Serving: Calories: 395; Total fat: 12g; Saturated fat: 2g; Cholesterol: 276mg; Sodium: 451mg; Carbohydrates: 41g; Fiber: 4g; Sugar: 5g; Protein: 45g

Honey-Walnut Shrimp

This isn't your average fast-food honey-walnut shrimp. The shrimp are coated in cornstarch and pan-fried until golden brown, then covered in a sweet, salty, and spicy glaze with crisp walnuts. It's much lighter than the traditional deep-fried version and includes several MIND diet foods.

FOR THE HONEY-WALNUT SAUCE

¼ cup unsalted vegetable stock

2 tablespoons evaporated milk

1 tablespoon cornstarch

¼ cup honey

3 tablespoons low-sodium soy sauce

▶ 2 garlic cloves, peeled and minced

1 teaspoon sriracha

▶ ½ cup chopped walnuts

FOR THE SHRIMP

▶ 1½ pounds shrimp, peeled, deveined and tails removed

½ cup cornstarch

½ teaspoon kosher or sea salt

▶ 3 tablespoons avocado oil

▶ 2 medium scallions, both white and green parts, thinly sliced

GLUTEN-FREE

Serves: 6

Prep Time: 15 to 20 minutes

Cook Time: 20 to 25 minutes

Cooking tip
If using frozen shrimp, remove them from the bag and place in a colander. Rinse them with cold water until thawed. Pat them dry with paper towel before using.

Variation tip
Try with thinly sliced boneless, skinless chicken breast.

1. To make the honey-walnut sauce, in a medium bowl, whisk together the stock, evaporated milk, and cornstarch until dissolved. Whisk in the honey, soy sauce, garlic, and sriracha. Fold in the walnuts. Set aside.

2. To make the shrimp, place them in a large bowl with a lid or in a large resealable plastic bag and add the cornstarch and salt. Shake until the shrimp are coated.

3. In a large nonstick sauté pan or skillet, heat the oil over medium-high heat. Once hot, add the shrimp, one at a time, and sauté for 1 to 2 minutes per side, until shrimp are browned and crispy. Pour the honey sauce into the skillet and stir. Bring to a simmer. Cook for 1 to 2 minutes, stirring constantly, until the sauce is thickened, and the shrimp tails have slightly curled in. Serve the shrimp with scallions on top.

4. The shrimp can be prepped in advance and stored in airtight containers for up to 3 days. Reheat by toasting under a low broil until crispy.

Per Serving: Calories: 331; Total fat: 14g; Saturated fat: 2g; Cholesterol: 185mg; Sodium: 553mg; Carbohydrates: 26g; Fiber: 1g; Sugar: 13g; Protein: 30g

Grilled Chimichurri Scallops

Grilling provides a depth of flavor to food that is hard to beat. And when doused with chimichurri sauce, a simple herb and garlic condiment, these scallops go from great to amazing. Sea or diver scallops are large and easy to grill, whereas bay scallops are small and better for pan-frying or broiling.

FOR THE CHIMICHURRI

½ cup fresh flat-leaf parsley

▶ 3 to 4 garlic cloves, peeled

¼ cup red wine vinegar

¼ cup fresh cilantro

▶ 2 tablespoons extra-virgin olive oil

▶ ½ medium jalapeño, seeded

1 teaspoon dried oregano leaves

½ teaspoon kosher or sea salt

¼ teaspoon freshly ground black pepper

FOR THE GRILLED SCALLOPS

▶ 1½ pounds sea or diver scallops, cleaned and patted dry

▶ 1 tablespoon extra-virgin olive oil

¼ teaspoon kosher or sea salt

¼ teaspoon freshly ground black pepper

DAIRY-FREE
GLUTEN-FREE
NUT-FREE

Serves: 4
Prep Time: 10 to 15 minutes
Cook Time: 5 to 10 minutes

Variation tip
Try salmon instead of scallops.

Cooking tip
Make this recipe indoors by using a stovetop grill pan over medium heat.

1. To make the chimichurri, in the bowl of a food processor, combine the parsley, garlic, vinegar, cilantro, olive oil, jalapeño, oregano, salt, and pepper and pulse until pesto-consistency is reached, scraping the sides of the bowl with a spatula as needed. Taste and adjust seasoning, if necessary. Refrigerate.

2. To make the grilled scallops, preheat the grill to medium. Rub the scallops with olive oil, then season with the salt and pepper. Place the scallops on the grill and cook for 2 to 3 minutes per side, until the scallops are firm. Serve topped with chimichurri sauce.

3. The chimichurri sauce can be prepped in advance and stored in airtight containers for up to 3 days in the refrigerator. The grilled scallops can be prepped in advance and stored in airtight containers for up to 2 days. Reheat by toasting scallops under a low broiler until crispy. Top grilled scallops with chimichurri just before serving.

Per Serving: Calories: 218; Total fat: 11g; Saturated fat: 2g; Cholesterol: 18mg; Sodium: 307mg; Carbohydrates: 7g; Fiber: 1g; Sugar: 0g; Protein: 21g

Crab Cake Bites with Dill Tartar Sauce

Crab cakes are fun, but crab cake bites are even better. They're perfect for dipping or served on top of a salad or in a veggie bowl. Crab is a great source of omega-3 fats and protein, so eat up!

FOR THE CRAB BITES

▸ 18 ounces cooked lump crab

½ cup panko bread crumbs

▸ 2 large eggs

2 tablespoons Dijon mustard

▸ 1 tablespoon extra-virgin olive oil

2 teaspoons dried oregano leaves

▸ Zest of ½ medium lemon (about 1 tablespoon each)

¾ teaspoon kosher or sea salt

½ teaspoon freshly ground black pepper

FOR THE DILL TARTAR SAUCE

▸ 2 tablespoons plain yogurt (not Greek)

2 tablespoons mayonnaise

1 tablespoon dill pickle relish

2 tablespoons chopped fresh dill (optional)

¼ teaspoon freshly ground black pepper

NUT-FREE

Serves: 4

Prep Time: 10 to 15 minutes

Cook Time: 12 to 15 minutes

Cooking tip
You can use canned, pouched, or imitation crab for this recipe.

Substitution tip
For a dairy-free version, use plain dairy-free yogurt.

1. Preheat the oven to 400°F. Fit a baking sheet with a wire rack and coat with cooking spray. Set aside.

2. To make the crab bites, in a medium bowl, mix together the crab, bread crumbs, eggs, mustard, olive oil, oregano, lemon zest, salt, and pepper until thoroughly combined. Roll the mixture into 2-inch bites and place on the prepared wire rack about 1 inch apart. Coat the bites with cooking spray. Bake for 12 to 15 minutes, or until the bites are set and lightly browned on the outside.

3. Meanwhile, to make the dill tartar sauce, in a small bowl, combine the yogurt, mayonnaise, relish, dill (if using), and pepper and stir. Taste and adjust seasoning, if necessary. Serve immediately with tartar sauce.

4. The crab cake bites can be prepped in advance and stored in airtight containers for up to 3 days. Reheat by toasting under a low broil until crispy. The tartar sauce can be prepped in advance and stored in an airtight container for up to 3 days in the refrigerator. Serve tartar sauce with crab cake bites.

Per Serving (3 bites): Calories: 240; Total fat: 12g; Saturated fat: 2g; Cholesterol: 218mg; Sodium: 494mg; Carbohydrates: 9g; Fiber: 1g; Sugar: 1g; Protein: 22g

Oven-"Fried" Calamari with Marinara

Squid is a good source of vitamin B$_{12}$, an important nutrient for brain health, and is low in saturated fat. It's typically served deep-fried as calamari, but I've developed a just-as-tasty version that is baked. The marinara we're serving it with is packed with vitamin C and folate. You can use premade marinara; just check the label and choose one with the lowest amount of sodium.

FOR THE MARINARA

- ▸ 1 tablespoon extra-virgin olive oil
- ▸ ½ medium yellow onion, peeled and minced
- ▸ 2 garlic cloves, peeled and minced
- 1½ teaspoons dried oregano leaves
- ¾ teaspoon kosher or sea salt
- ▸ 1 (15-ounce) can no-salt-added, crushed tomatoes
- 1 teaspoon granulated sugar

FOR THE OVEN-"FRIED" CALAMARI

- ½ cup all-purpose or whole-wheat flour
- ▸ 2 large eggs
- 2 cups panko bread crumbs
- 2 tablespoons Italian seasoning
- 1 teaspoon kosher or sea salt, divided
- ½ teaspoon freshly ground black pepper, divided
- ▸ 1 pound squid rings

DAIRY-FREE
NUT-FREE

Serves: 4
Prep Time: 10 to 15 minutes
Cook Time: 15 to 20 minutes

Cooking tip
Squid rings are typically available in the frozen section of the grocery store or can be found fresh at most seafood markets.

Substitution tip
Use gluten-free panko bread crumbs for a gluten-free version.

1. Preheat the oven to 400°F. Place a wire rack inside a baking sheet and coat with cooking spray.

2. In a large saucepan, heat the olive oil over medium heat. Add the onion and sauté for 4 to 5 minutes, or until the onions are soft. Stir in the garlic, oregano, and salt and sauté for 30 to 60 seconds, or until fragrant. Add the crushed tomatoes and bring to a simmer for 10 to 15 minutes, or until slightly thickened. Stir in the sugar. Taste and adjust seasoning, if necessary.

3. Meanwhile, set up three bowls: one with flour, one with beaten egg, and one with panko bread crumbs and Italian seasoning. Divide salt and pepper between the bowls and stir each to combine.

4. Working one at a time, dip the calamari rings into the flour, then the egg, then the bread crumb mixture and line up on the prepared wire rack. Coat each with cooking spray. Bake for 10 to 15 minutes, or until the calamari rings are firm and the breading is browned and crisp. Serve immediately with marinara.

5. The marinara can be prepped in advance and stored in airtight containers for up to 4 days in the refrigerator. The calamari can be prepped in advance and stored in airtight containers for up to 2 days. Reheat by toasting under a low broil until crispy. Serve calamari with marinara.

Per Serving: Calories: 280; Total fat: 6g; Saturated fat: 1g; Cholesterol: 93mg; Sodium: 240mg; Carbohydrates: 44g; Fiber: 5g; Sugar: 7g; Protein: 10g

Easy Seafood Paella

Paella is a seafood-loaded Spanish rice dish that is made with saffron; the stigmas of crocus flowers that give paella its signature flavor and hue. If you aren't able to find saffron, you can skip it, but it truly is worth splurging on if you want to try something new or maintain authenticity.

4½ cups unsalted vegetable or seafood stock, divided

1 teaspoon Spanish saffron (optional)

▸ 3 tablespoons extra-virgin olive oil

▸ ½ medium yellow onion, peeled and diced

3 ounces ground Spanish chorizo (optional)

▸ 3 cups baby spinach leaves or chopped kale

▸ 3 garlic cloves, peeled and minced

1½ teaspoons kosher or sea salt

1 teaspoon sweet or smoked paprika

½ teaspoon freshly ground black pepper

▸ 2 cups brown rice

▸ 1 (15-ounce) can no-salt-added, fire-roasted diced tomatoes, drained

▸ 1 cup frozen peas

▸ 1 pound large shrimp, peeled and deveined

▸ 8 ounces mussels, scrubbed and rinsed

▸ Zest and juice of 1 medium lemon (about 2 tablespoons each) (optional)

½ cup chopped fresh flat-leaf Italian parsley (optional)

DAIRY-FREE
GLUTEN-FREE
NUT-FREE

Serves: 8
Prep Time: 15 to 20 minutes
Cook Time: 60 to 70 minutes

Cooking tip
For a spicy version, add ½ teaspoon red pepper flakes. Store saffron in a cool, dry, dark place.

Variation tip
Try this dish with bay scallops and clams.

1. In a small bowl, combine ½ cup of the stock and the saffron strands (if using). Set aside and let sit for 5 minutes.

2. In a Dutch oven, heat the olive oil over medium heat. Add the onion and chorizo (if using) and sauté for 4 to 5 minutes, or until the onions are soft. Add the spinach, garlic, salt, paprika, and pepper and sauté for 30 to 60 seconds, or until fragrant. Stir in the rice, tomatoes, peas, the remaining 4 cups of stock, and the saffron with its soaking liquid and bring to a simmer.

3. Place a lid on the pot and let simmer for 35 to 40 minutes, stirring occasionally. Add the shrimp and mussels, place a lid on the pot, and cook for another 10 to 15 minutes, or until the mussels have opened and the shrimp are slightly firm. Stir in the lemon zest and juice (if using) and parsley (if using). Taste and adjust seasoning, if necessary. Serve.

4. The paella can be prepped in advance and stored in airtight containers for up to 3 days in the refrigerator. Reheat the paella in the microwave for 2 to 3 minutes or until heated through.

Per Serving: Calories: 387; Total fat: 7g; Saturated fat: 1g; Cholesterol: 100mg; Sodium: 481mg; Carbohydrates: 56g; Fiber: 5g; Sugar: 13g; Protein: 27g

Jerk Pork Tacos with Pineapple Salsa, Page 136

CHAPTER EIGHT

Carnivore Mains

Sweet-and-Sour Chicken

Poultry is one of the featured MIND diet foods because it contains B vitamins, which we know are important for brain health. There are numerous ways to cook chicken, but one of my favorites is to make healthier sweet-and-sour chicken. This version has a tangy pineapple sauce with chunks of crispy chicken, fresh pineapple, and bell peppers.

FOR THE SWEET-AND-SOUR SAUCE

1¼ cups 100 percent pineapple juice

1 tablespoon cornstarch

2 tablespoons apple cider vinegar

2 tablespoons low sodium ketchup

1 tablespoon granulated sugar

FOR THE CHICKEN

▸ 3 tablespoons avocado oil, divided

▸ 1 medium red bell pepper, cubed

▸ 1 pound boneless, skinless chicken breast, cubed

¼ cup cornstarch

¾ teaspoon kosher or sea salt

▸ ½ medium pineapple, peeled, cored, and diced (about 5 cups)

▸ 2 medium scallions, thinly sliced, both green and white parts (optional)

DAIRY-FREE
GLUTEN-FREE
NUT-FREE

Serves: 4

Prep Time: 15 to 20 minutes

Cook Time: 20 to 25 minutes

Substitution tip
Try this with tofu for a meatless dish.

Variation tip
Use a mix of boneless, skinless thigh and breast meat.

1. To make the sweet-and-sour sauce, in a medium saucepan, whisk together the pineapple juice and cornstarch until dissolved. Whisk in the vinegar, ketchup, and sugar. Bring to a simmer for 2 to 3 minutes, or until thickened, whisking constantly. Set aside.

2. To make the chicken, in a large nonstick sauté pan or skillet, heat 1 tablespoon of the oil over medium heat. Add the bell pepper and sauté for 2 to 3 minutes, or until slightly soft. Remove from the skillet and set aside.

3. Place the chicken in a large bowl. Add the cornstarch and salt, place a lid on top of the bowl and shake until the chicken is coated (or use a large resealable plastic bag).

4. In the same large skillet, heat the remaining 2 tablespoons of oil over medium heat. Working in batches, add the chicken and sauté for 5 to 7 minutes, stirring occasionally, until all sides are browned and crisp. Remove the chicken from the pan and set aside as you cook the remaining chicken.

5. Place all of the chicken back in the skillet or wok and coat with the sweet-and-sour sauce. Fold in the bell pepper and pineapple. Serve garnished with scallions (if using).

6. The sweet-and-sour chicken can be prepped in advance and stored in airtight containers up to 3 days in the refrigerator. Reheat by toasting under a broiler set to low until crispy or microwave for 2 to 3 minutes, or until heated through.

Per Serving: Calories: 408; Total fat: 17g; Saturated fat: 2g; Cholesterol: 73mg; Sodium: 379mg; Carbohydrates: 37g; Fiber: 5g; Sugar: 23g; Protein: 26g

Cornmeal-Crusted Chicken Tenders

Serving chicken tenders for dinner is a surefire way to make the entire family happy. By coating them in a mixture of cornmeal and spices, these tenders get extra crispy and have stellar flavor. I like to serve them with yogurt ranch dressing and a green salad.

½ cup all-purpose or whole-wheat flour

▸ 2 large eggs, beaten

½ cup buttermilk

▸ 2 cups cornmeal

1½ teaspoons kosher or sea salt, divided

1 teaspoon freshly ground black pepper, divided

1 teaspoon onion powder, divided

1 teaspoon garlic powder, divided

1 teaspoon smoked paprika, divided

½ teaspoon ground cayenne pepper, divided

▸ 1½ pounds boneless skinless chicken breasts, cut into tenders

NUT-FREE

Serves: 6

Prep Time: 10 to 15 minutes

Cook Time: 10 to 15 minutes

Cooking tip
If you don't have buttermilk, use ½ cup milk mixed with 1 tablespoon white or apple cider vinegar.

Substitution tip
Use gluten-free all-purpose flour for a gluten-free version.

1. Preheat the oven to 375°F. Fit a wire rack inside a baking sheet and coat with cooking spray. Set aside.

2. Set up three bowls: one with flour, one with beaten egg and buttermilk, and one with cornmeal. Divide the salt, pepper, onion powder, garlic powder, smoked paprika, and cayenne pepper between the bowls and stir each to combine.

3. Working one at a time, dip the chicken tenders into the flour, then the egg, then the cornmeal and arrange on the prepared wire rack. Coat each with cooking spray. Bake for 10 to 15 minutes, or until chicken tenders are firm. Serve immediately.

4. The chicken tenders can be prepped in advance and stored in airtight containers for up to 4 days in the refrigerator. Reheat by toasting under a low broil until crispy.

Per Serving: Calories: 339; Total fat: 5g; Saturated fat: 1g; Cholesterol: 136mg; Sodium: 459mg; Carbohydrates: 41g; Fiber: 2g; Sugar: 2g; Protein: 31g

Barbecue Spice–Roasted Chicken Legs

Once you make your own barbecue spice rub, you'll want to keep a jar of it in the refrigerator to use on everything. It hits all the right notes—sweet, spicy, and savory—and goes perfectly with chicken. These chicken legs are rubbed, then roasted, but you could also grill them and serve with potato salad or coleslaw for an easy summer meal.

FOR THE BARBECUE SPICE RUB

1 tablespoon sweet or smoked paprika

1 teaspoon dark brown sugar

1 teaspoon chili powder

1 teaspoon garlic powder

1 teaspoon onion powder

1 teaspoon freshly ground black pepper

1 teaspoon kosher or sea salt

¼ teaspoon ground cayenne pepper

FOR THE CHICKEN LEGS

▸ 1 pound chicken legs

▸ 2 tablespoons avocado oil

DAIRY-FREE
GLUTEN-FREE
NUT-FREE

Serves: 6
Prep Time: 10 to 15 minutes
Cook Time: 25 to 30 minutes

Cooking tip
Store excess spice rub in an airtight container in the refrigerator.

Variation tip
Try this recipe with chicken breasts or thighs.

1. Preheat the oven to 400°F. Fit a wire rack into a baking sheet and coat with cooking spray. Set aside.

2. To make the barbecue spice rub, in a small bowl, whisk together the paprika, brown sugar, chili powder, garlic powder, onion powder, pepper, salt, and cayenne pepper.

3. To make the chicken legs, rub the chicken legs with oil, then the spice rub. Place them on the prepared baking sheet. Roast for 15 to 20 minutes, then switch the oven to broil. Broil for 5 to 6 minutes, using tongs to turn the legs halfway through, or until the skin on all sides is browned and crispy and juices run clear. Test for doneness by inserting an instant-read thermometer into the thickest part of the chicken leg; it should reach an internal temperature of 165°F. Remove from the oven and let rest 5 minutes; serve.

4. The chicken legs can be prepped in advance and stored in airtight containers for up to 4 days in the refrigerator. Reheat in the microwave for 2 to 3 minutes, or until heated through.

Per Serving: Calories: 294; Total fat: 8g; Saturated fat: 2g; Cholesterol: 41mg; Sodium: 575mg; Carbohydrates: 28g; Fiber: 5g; Sugar: 4g; Protein: 25g

Spanish Chicken Skillet

This is my favorite chicken dish to prepare on a Sunday afternoon because it makes my house smell wonderful and I only dirty one pot. It is loaded with MIND diet foods, has a ton of color, and is filled with flavorful herbs and spices. Basically, it's everything you could ever want in a casserole.

- 2 tablespoons extra-virgin olive oil
- 1½ pounds boneless or bone-in chicken thighs, skin-on or skinless
- 1 medium yellow onion, peeled and diced
- 4 cups baby spinach leaves or chopped kale
- 3 garlic cloves, peeled and minced
- 2 medium Yukon Gold or red potatoes, diced
- 2 teaspoons Italian seasoning
- 1½ teaspoons sweet or smoked paprika

- 1½ teaspoons kosher or sea salt
- 1 teaspoon ground cumin
- ½ teaspoon freshly ground black pepper
- 1 (28-ounce) can no-salt-added, crushed tomatoes
- 1½ cups unsalted chicken stock
- Zest and juice of 1 medium lemon (about 2 tablespoons each)
- ½ cup chopped fresh cilantro (optional)

DAIRY-FREE
GLUTEN-FREE
NUT-FREE

Serves: 6
Prep Time: 10 to 15 minutes
Cook Time: 25 to 30 minutes

Cooking tip
Be sure the pot is hot before adding the chicken to it. This ensures that the chicken won't stick to the bottom and it'll get a crispier crust.

Variation tip
Add ½ cup pitted green olives for a bit more flavor.

1. In a shallow Dutch oven or stovetop casserole dish, heat the olive oil over medium heat. Add the chicken thighs and cook for 2 to 3 minutes per side, or until browned and crispy. Remove and set aside.

2. Add the onion and sauté for 4 to 5 minutes, or until soft. Stir in the spinach and garlic and sauté for 2 to 3 minutes, until the greens are wilted.

3. Stir in the potatoes, Italian seasoning, paprika, salt, cumin, and pepper. Add the chicken, tomatoes, stock, and lemon zest and juice and bring to a simmer. Cover and cook for 15 to 20 minutes, or until potatoes are *al dente* and the chicken is fully cooked, stirring occasionally.

4. Stir in the cilantro (if using). Taste and adjust seasoning, if necessary. Serve immediately.

5. The Spanish chicken can be prepped in advance and stored in airtight containers for up to 4 days in the refrigerator. Reheat in the microwave for 2 to 3 minutes, or until heated through.

Per Serving: Calories: 492; Total fat: 15g; Saturated fat: 1g; Cholesterol: 110mg; Sodium: 567mg; Carbohydrates: 54g; Fiber: 10g; Sugar: 27g; Protein: 32g

Chicken Caesar Salad Pizza

If you're going to make homemade pizza, why not throw some Caesar salad on top? The crust is impossibly crispy because it's made with Greek yogurt (odd, but true), the pizza sauce is now Caesar dressing, and it's all topped with juicy chicken, a little mozzarella cheese, and handfuls of Caesar salad. It's so good (and yes, MIND diet compliant!).

FOR THE PIZZA CRUST

- 1¾ cup whole-wheat flour, plus more for dusting
- 1⅓ cups plain Greek yogurt

1 teaspoon baking soda

¼ teaspoon kosher or sea salt

- 1 tablespoon extra-virgin olive oil

FOR THE PIZZA

⅓ cup Caesar dressing, divided

- 8 ounces cooked chicken breast, sliced

½ cup shredded mozzarella cheese

- 2 heads romaine lettuce, thinly sliced

¼ cup freshly shaved Parmesan cheese

NUT-FREE

Serves: 6

Prep Time: 10 to 15 minutes

Cook Time: 25 to 30 minutes

Substitution tip
For a gluten-free pizza, use gluten-free all-purpose flour to make the crust.

Cooking tip
To make your own Caesar dressing, whisk together ¼ cup olive oil, 2 tablespoons mayonnaise, 2 tablespoons freshly grated Parmesan, 1 teaspoon anchovy paste, 2 minced garlic cloves, zest and juice of ½ medium lemon, 2 teaspoons Worcestershire sauce, 1 teaspoon granulated sugar, ½ teaspoon freshly ground black pepper, and ¼ teaspoon kosher or sea salt.

1. Preheat the oven to 400°F. Coat a round, 15-inch pizza pan with cooking spray. Set aside.

2. To make the pizza crust, in a large bowl, stir together the flour, yogurt, baking soda, and salt until well combined. Transfer the mixture to a floured cutting board. Work the dough with your hands and press out into a circle the size of the pizza pan. Transfer to the prepared pizza pan. Brush dough with the olive oil. Bake for 7 to 8 minutes or until crust is starting to brown.

3. To make the pizza, spread half of the Caesar dressing onto the pre-baked crust in a thin layer. Cover with the cooked chicken breast strips and sprinkle with mozzarella cheese. Bake for an additional 5 to 6 minutes, or until the crust is golden brown and the cheese is bubbly.

4. Meanwhile, in a medium bowl, toss the remaining Caesar dressing with the romaine lettuce and Parmesan cheese until coated. Top pizza with Caesar salad, slice, and serve immediately.

5. Once the Caesar salad is on top of the pizza, reheating is not recommended. Prepare the pizza just before serving.

Per Serving: Calories: 294; Total fat: 8g; Saturated fat: 2g; Cholesterol: 41mg; Sodium: 575mg; Carbohydrates: 28g; Fiber: 5g; Sugar: 4g; Protein: 25g

Curried Turkey and Grape Lettuce Wraps

Lettuce wraps have become a staple in my kitchen because they're an easy way to get in an extra serving of leafy green vegetables. This curry turkey and grape salad is also a staple because I can whip it up in a few minutes using leftover cooked turkey or chicken and it includes handfuls of fresh vegetables and fruit.

- ▸ ½ cup plain Greek yogurt
- 3 tablespoons mayonnaise
- ▸ Zest and juice of 1 medium lime (about 2 tablespoons each)
- 1 tablespoon honey
- 1 tablespoon curry powder
- ½ teaspoon kosher or sea salt
- ¼ teaspoon freshly ground black pepper
- ▸ 1½ cups chopped cooked turkey or chicken breast

- ▸ 1½ cups halved seedless grapes
- ▸ 1 medium English cucumber, diced
- ¼ cup fresh chopped cilantro (optional)
- ▸ ½ medium jalapeño, seeded and minced
- ▸ 1 head bibb or Boston lettuce, leaves separated
- ▸ ¼ cup chopped cashews (optional)

GLUTEN-FREE

Serves: 4

Prep Time: 10 to 15 minutes

Cooking tip
For a deeper flavor and crunchier texture, toast the cashews in a hot, dry skillet for 30 to 60 seconds.

Variation tip
For an extra serving of whole grains, stir ½ cup cooked quinoa or brown rice into the turkey salad.

1. In a large bowl, whisk together the yogurt, mayonnaise, lime zest and juice, honey, curry powder, salt, and pepper. Fold in the cooked turkey, grapes, cucumber, cilantro (if using), and jalapeño. Taste and adjust seasoning, if necessary. Refrigerate at least 30 minutes.

2. Scoop salad into bibb or Boston lettuce cups. Top with cashews (if using). Serve immediately.

3. The turkey salad can be prepped in advance and stored in airtight containers for up to 4 days in the refrigerator. Scoop into lettuce cups just before serving.

Per Serving: Calories: 247; Total fat: 10g; Saturated fat: 2g; Cholesterol: 51mg; Sodium: 269mg; Carbohydrates: 20g; Fiber: 4g; Sugar: 12g; Protein: 22g

Sheet-Pan Turkey Sausage, Potatoes, and Bell Peppers

While processed meats are not regularly recommended on the MIND diet, choosing a lower-fat, uncured sausage is a reasonable choice. It imparts a ton of flavor to the dish, and goes well with potatoes, bell peppers, and Italian seasoning. The fact that this is a sheet-pan meal also makes dinner prep simple and quick.

8 ounces uncured turkey or chicken smoked sausage, sliced

▸ 1 pound baby Yukon Gold or red potatoes, quartered

▸ 2 medium bell peppers, sliced

▸ 3 tablespoons extra-virgin olive oil

1 tablespoon Italian seasoning

½ teaspoon kosher or sea salt

½ teaspoon freshly ground black pepper

¼ teaspoon red pepper flakes

DAIRY-FREE
GLUTEN-FREE
NUT-FREE

Serves: 4
Prep Time: 10 to 15 minutes
Cook Time: 30 to 35 minutes

Cooking tip
Regular-size potatoes also work well for this dish; simply chop them into bite-size pieces.

Variation tip
Change up the veggies for something different. Try broccoli florets and mushrooms instead of bell peppers.

1. Preheat the oven to 400°F. Coat a baking sheet with cooking spray.

2. On the baking sheet, place the smoked sausage, potatoes, and bell peppers. Drizzle with olive oil and sprinkle with Italian seasoning, salt, pepper, and red pepper flakes. Toss to evenly coat. Roast for 30 to 35 minutes, or until the potatoes are tender and sausage and vegetables are lightly browned. Serve immediately.

3. The sheet-pan meal can be prepped in advance and stored in airtight containers for up to 4 days in the refrigerator. Reheat in the microwave for 2 to 3 minutes, or until heated through.

Per Serving: Calories: 305; Total fat: 16g; Saturated fat: 3g; Cholesterol: 30mg; Sodium: 614mg; Carbohydrates: 31g; Fiber: 5g; Sugar: 6g; Protein: 12g

Cheesy Slow Cooker Turkey Meatballs

Slow cooker meals make life so much easier during the week. These meatballs can be prepped in advance and tossed into the slow cooker before work and Voilà! Dinner is ready when you get home. This recipe also boasts several cups of leafy greens.

- 2 pounds ground turkey
- ⅓ cup panko bread crumbs
- 2 large eggs
- 2 tablespoons freshly grated Parmesan cheese
- 3 garlic cloves, peeled and minced
- 2 tablespoons Italian seasoning
- 1 tablespoon Dijon mustard
- 1 tablespoon minced onion
- 1 teaspoon kosher or sea salt
- ½ teaspoon freshly ground black pepper
- ¼ teaspoon red pepper flakes (optional)
- 2 (24-ounce) jars low-sodium marinara
- 4 cups baby spinach leaves or chopped kale
- ½ cup shredded mozzarella cheese (optional)

NUT-FREE

Serves: 8
Prep Time: 10 to 15 minutes
Cook Time: 2 to 3 hours

Cooking tip
To make the meatballs in the oven, bake on a greased wire rack at 400°F for 15 to 18 minutes. Serve with marinara and a green salad.

Variation tip
Serve over cooked, whole-grain pasta.

1. In a medium bowl, combine the ground turkey, bread crumbs, eggs, Parmesan, garlic, Italian seasoning, mustard, minced onion, salt, pepper, and red pepper flakes (if using). Form the mixture into 2-inch balls and place in the bowl of the slow cooker.

2. Add the marinara and spinach to the slow cooker and stir to combine. Cook on low for 4 to 5 hours or high for 2 to 3 hours. Sprinkle the cheese (if using), on top and cook for an additional 15 to 20 minutes, or until cheese is melted. Serve immediately.

3. The meatballs and sauce can be prepped in advance and stored in airtight containers for up to 4 days in the refrigerator. Reheat in the microwave for 2 to 3 minutes, or until heated through.

Per Serving: Calories: 310; Total fat: 18g; Saturated fat: 4g; Cholesterol: 131mg; Sodium: 509mg; Carbohydrates: 9g; Fiber: 2g; Sugar: 3g; Protein: 28g

Chipotle-Orange Pork Chops

I've said this many times, but sweet and spicy ingredients go well together, just like the orange and chipotle in this recipe. The cornstarch thickens the glaze, so it wraps itself around the seared pork chop like a blanket.

FOR THE PORK CHOPS

▸ 1 tablespoon avocado oil

1 pound bone-in or boneless, thick-cut pork chops

½ teaspoon kosher or sea salt

½ teaspoon freshly ground black pepper

FOR THE CHIPOTLE-ORANGE GLAZE

▸ Zest and juice of 2 medium oranges (about ½ cup each)

1 teaspoon cornstarch

1 tablespoon honey

1 chipotle chile in adobo sauce, chopped

DAIRY-FREE
GLUTEN-FREE
NUT-FREE

Serves: 4
Prep Time: 10 to 15 minutes
Cook Time: 10 to 15 minutes

Substitution tip
Try this recipe with chicken thighs or pork tenderloin.

Cooking tip
Let the pork chops sit at room temperature for 15 minutes before cooking, so they come to room temperature and cook evenly throughout. Bone-in pork chops will take a bit longer to cook than boneless.

1. To make the pork chops, in a large sauté pan or skillet, heat the oil over medium heat. Season the pork chops with the salt and pepper. Place the pork chops in the skillet and cook for 4 to 5 minutes per side, until each side is browned and crisp. Remove from the skillet and set aside.

2. To make the chipotle-orange glaze, in a small bowl, whisk together the orange zest and juice with the cornstarch until dissolved. Whisk in the honey and chipotle chile. Add the mixture to the hot skillet and whisk for 1 to 2 minutes, until thickened. Put the pork chops back in the skillet and cook for 2 to 3 minutes in the glaze, or until an instant-read thermometer inserted into the thickest part of the pork chops reaches 145°F.

3. Serve the pork chops on plates and spoon the glaze over the top.

4. The pork chops with the glaze can be prepped in advance and stored in airtight containers for up to 3 days in the refrigerator. Reheat in the microwave for 1 to 2 minutes, or until heated through.

Per Serving: Calories: 256; Total fat: 12g; Saturated fat: 3g; Cholesterol: 75mg; Sodium: 225mg; Carbohydrates: 13g; Fiber: 2g; Sugar: 12g; Protein: 25g

Jerk Pork Tacos with Pineapple Salsa

Tacos aren't just for Tuesdays. The salsa is loaded with vitamin C and its cool juiciness makes it the perfect topping for the jerk pork tacos with creamy avocado. You could substitute chicken breast or use ground pork, turkey, or chicken, if that's what you have on hand.

FOR THE PINEAPPLE SALSA

▸ ½ medium pineapple, peeled and diced (about 1½ cups)

▸ ¼ medium red onion, peeled and minced

¼ cup chopped fresh cilantro

▸ Zest and juice of 1 medium lime (about 1 tablespoon each)

▸ ½ medium jalapeño, seeded and minced

¼ teaspoon kosher or sea salt

FOR THE JERK TACOS

▸ 1 tablespoon extra-virgin olive oil

1 pound boneless pork chops or tenderloin, cubed

1 tablespoon jerk seasoning

½ teaspoon kosher or sea salt

¼ teaspoon freshly ground black pepper

▸ 8 corn tortillas, toasted

▸ 1 medium avocado, peeled, pitted, and sliced

▸ 1 medium lime, cut into wedges (optional)

DAIRY-FREE
GLUTEN-FREE
NUT-FREE

Serves: 4
Prep Time: 10 to 15 minutes
Cook Time: 10 to 15 minutes

Substitution tip
To make your own salt-free jerk seasoning, combine 3 tablespoons sweet paprika, 3 tablespoons garlic powder, 1 tablespoon ground allspice, 1½ teaspoons ground nutmeg, and ½ teaspoon cayenne pepper. Store the excess in an airtight container up to 2 months.

Cooking tip
Toast corn tortillas in a hot, dry skillet until lightly browned on both sides.

1. To make the pineapple salsa, in a medium bowl, stir together the pineapple, onion, cilantro, lime zest and juice, jalapeño, and salt. Taste and adjust seasoning, if necessary.

2. To make the jerk tacos, in a large sauté pan or skillet, heat the olive oil over medium heat. Dust the pork with the jerk seasoning, salt, and pepper. Add the pork to the skillet and sauté for 4 to 5 minutes, stirring occasionally, until the pork is lightly browned on all sides and the pork cubes are firm.

3. Serve the pork in toasted corn tortillas with sliced avocado, pineapple salsa, and lime wedges (if using).

4. The jerk pork can be prepped in advance and stored in airtight containers for up to 3 days in the refrigerator. Reheat in the microwave for 1 to 2 minutes, or until heated through. The pineapple salsa can be prepped in advance and stored in airtight containers for up to 3 days in the refrigerator. Assemble tacos just before serving.

Per Serving (2 tacos): Calories: 363; Total fat: 13g; Saturated fat: 2g; Cholesterol: 60mg; Sodium: 286mg; Carbohydrates: 39g; Fiber: 8g; Sugar: 11g; Protein: 27g

Spicy Pork Noodle Bowls

Noodle bowls are a great way to cook with a wide variety of vegetables. I like to use vegetables with several different colors to get the most nutrition out of them. I also like to use brown rice noodles rather than ramen because they are a good source of fiber.

- 1 tablespoon avocado oil

  1 pound lean ground pork
- 1 cup shredded carrots
- 1 cup shredded green or purple cabbage
- 2-inch piece fresh ginger, peeled and minced
- 4 garlic cloves, peeled and minced

  1 teaspoon kosher or sea salt

  8 cups unsalted chicken or vegetable stock

  ¼ cup low-sodium soy sauce

  1 tablespoon dark brown sugar
- 1½ teaspoons sesame oil

  1½ teaspoons sriracha
- 8 ounces brown rice noodles
- Zest and juice of 1 medium lime (about 1 tablespoon each) (optional)

  ½ cup chopped fresh cilantro or 2 medium scallions, thinly sliced (optional)
- ½ cup chopped roasted peanuts (optional)

DAIRY-FREE

Serves: 8
Prep Time: 10 to 15 minutes
Cook Time: 15 to 20 minutes

Substitution tip
Try ground turkey or chicken instead of pork.

Variation tip
Add sliced mushrooms, sliced bok choy, or pea pods for a boost of veggies.

1. In a shallow Dutch oven or stovetop casserole dish, heat the oil over medium heat. Add the pork and sauté for 3 to 4 minutes, breaking the pork up with a wooden spoon as it cooks.

2. Add the carrots and cabbage and sauté for another 3 to 4 minutes, until the pork is fully cooked and the vegetables are slightly soft. Stir in the ginger, garlic, and salt and sauté for 30 to 60 seconds, until the garlic is fragrant.

3. Add the stock, soy sauce, brown sugar, sesame oil, and sriracha and bring to a simmer. Add the noodles and cook for 7 to 8 minutes, until the noodles are soft, adding more stock if desired. Stir in the lime zest and juice (if using). Taste the broth and adjust seasoning, if necessary.

4. Serve in bowls topped with cilantro (if using) and peanuts (if using).

5. The noodle bowls can be prepped in advance and stored in airtight containers for up to 3 days in the refrigerator. Reheat in the microwave for 1 to 2 minutes, or until heated through.

Per Serving: Calories: 317; Total fat: 15g; Saturated fat: 5g; Cholesterol: 40mg; Sodium: 592mg; Carbohydrates: 30g; Fiber: 2g; Sugar: 4g; Protein: 19g

Beef and Butternut Squash Tagine

Great news! You can still enjoy your favorite beef dishes while following the MIND diet. Beef may be a "sometimes food" on the MIND diet, but lean cuts of beef like tenderloin are lower in saturated fat than other cuts. As you can see, this dish only has 1 gram of saturated fat per serving.

- 1 tablespoon avocado oil
- 1 tablespoon ground cinnamon
- 2 teaspoons sweet or smoked paprika
- 1½ teaspoons kosher or sea salt
- 1 teaspoon ground cumin
- ½ teaspoon freshly ground black pepper
- 1 pound beef tenderloin, trimmed and cubed
- ½ medium yellow onion, peeled and diced
- 2-inch piece fresh ginger, peeled and minced

- 3 garlic cloves, peeled and minced
- ½ medium butternut squash, peeled and cubed (about 4 cups)
- 3½ cups unsalted beef stock
- 1 (15-ounce) can no-salt-added, fire-roasted diced tomatoes, drained
- ½ cup chopped fresh cilantro
- ¼ cup chopped roasted peanuts (optional)

DAIRY-FREE
GLUTEN-FREE

Serves: 6
Prep Time: 15 to 20 minutes
Cook Time: 25 to 30 minutes

Cooking tip
Add a pinch of cayenne pepper or red pepper flakes for a spicy version.

Variation tip
Try sweet potatoes instead of butternut squash.

1. In a Dutch oven or stock pot, heat the oil over medium heat.
2. In a small bowl, whisk together the cinnamon, paprika, salt, cumin, and pepper. Dust half of the mixture on the cubed beef and toss to coat. Add the beef to the pot and sauté for 1 to 2 minutes per side, or until lightly browned. Using tongs, remove the beef and set aside.

3. Add the onion to the pot and sauté for 4 to 5 minutes, or until soft. Add the ginger, garlic, and remaining spice mixture and sauté for 30 to 60 seconds, or until fragrant. Stir in the butternut squash and beef.

4. Add the stock and diced tomatoes and bring to a low simmer. Cover and cook for 15 to 20 minutes, stirring occasionally, until the butternut squash is tender and the beef is cooked through. Stir in the cilantro. Taste and adjust seasoning, if necessary.

5. Serve tagine in bowls topped with peanuts (if using). Serve immediately.

6. The tagine can be prepped in advance and stored in airtight containers up to 3 days in the refrigerator. Reheat in the micro-wave 2 to 3 minutes, or until heated through.

Per Serving: Calories: 388; Total fat: 7g; Saturated fat: 1g; Cholesterol: 40mg; Sodium: 540mg; Carbohydrates: 55g; Fiber: 9g; Sugar: 26g; Protein: 27g

Beef and Zucchini Lasagna Rolls

While whole-grain pasta is part of the MIND diet, this zucchini version is an easy way to get in several servings of vegetables in one sitting. In place of lasagna noodles, you use thin slices of zucchini. Zucchini contains vitamin C, folate, and vitamin B$_6$ and if you're a gardener, you're likely looking for some fun ways to use it up.

- 5 medium zucchinis, thinly sliced lengthwise
- 1½ teaspoons kosher or sea salt, divided
- 1 tablespoon extra-virgin olive oil
- ½ medium yellow onion, peeled and diced
- 1 pound lean ground beef
- 2 cups baby spinach leaves or chopped kale
- 3 garlic cloves, peeled and minced

- 1 cup ricotta cheese
- 2 large eggs
- 1½ tablespoons Italian seasoning
- ½ teaspoon freshly ground black pepper
- 24 ounces low-sodium marinara
- ½ cup shredded mozzarella cheese
- ¼ cup fresh basil chiffonade (optional)

GLUTEN-FREE
NUT-FREE

Serves: 6
Prep Time: 15 to 20 minutes
Cook Time: 25 to 30 minutes

Substitution tip
Try with ground turkey or chicken instead of beef.

Cooking tip
Use a vegetable peeler to thinly slice the zucchinis lengthwise.

1. Preheat the oven to 375°F.
2. Lay the zucchini slices out on a baking sheet or cutting board and sprinkle with ½ teaspoon salt. Let sit 10 minutes, then pat dry with paper towel. Set aside.
3. In the meantime, in a shallow Dutch oven or large oven-safe, nonstick sauté pan or skillet, heat the olive oil over medium heat. Add the onion and sauté for 4 to 5 minutes, then add the ground beef and spinach and sauté for an additional 6 to 7 minutes, until the beef is browned, breaking up the beef with a wooden spoon as it cooks. Add the garlic and sauté for 30 to 60 seconds, until fragrant. Drain any excess fat from the beef mixture, then transfer to a large mixing bowl.

4. To the bowl, add the ricotta, eggs, Italian seasoning, remaining 1 teaspoon salt, and pepper and stir to thoroughly combine. Set aside.

5. Pour the marinara into the same Dutch oven.

6. Stack two slices of zucchini on top of each other, then dollop a tablespoon of the ricotta mixture onto the middle of the top slice. Tightly roll the zucchini around the ricotta mixture, as if you were rolling lasagna noodles around the filling, then place in the pot with the marinara. Repeat with the remaining zucchini slices and ricotta mixture, lining them up in the pan until it is filled.

7. Top the zucchini rolls with shredded mozzarella cheese. Bake for 25 to 30 minutes, until the cheese is lightly browned and bubbly. Top with fresh basil (if using) and serve immediately.

8. The zucchini rolls can be prepped in advance and stored in airtight containers for up to 4 days in the refrigerator. Reheat in the microwave for 2 to 3 minutes or until heated through.

Per Serving: Calories: 335; Total fat: 19g; Saturated fat: 5g; Cholesterol: 126mg; Sodium: 582mg; Carbohydrates: 13g; Fiber: 3g; Sugar: 5g; Protein: 27g

Mongolian Beef and Vegetables

I adore a good stir-fry dish that takes less than 30 minutes to make. I generally keep soy sauce, sesame oil, ginger, and garlic on hand so I can use up any leftover vegetables for that evening's concoction.

FOR THE MONGOLIAN SAUCE

¼ cup unsalted beef stock

1 tablespoon cornstarch

¼ cup low-sodium soy sauce

1 tablespoon dark brown sugar

▶ 1 teaspoon sesame oil

FOR THE MONGOLIAN BEEF

12 ounces beef flank steak, thinly sliced

2 tablespoons cornstarch

¼ teaspoon kosher or sea salt

▶ 2 tablespoons avocado oil

▶ 2 medium carrots, peeled and thinly sliced

▶ 1 cup snow peas, halved

▶ ½ medium yellow onion, peeled and thinly sliced

▶ 1-inch piece fresh ginger, peeled and minced

▶ 3 garlic cloves, peeled and minced

▶ 2 medium scallions, both green and white parts, thinly sliced (optional)

DAIRY-FREE
NUT-FREE

Serves: 4
Prep Time: 15 to 20 minutes
Cook Time: 15 to 20 minutes

Cooking tip
Store fresh ginger root in a sealed plastic bag in the refrigerator up to 2 months.

Variation tip
Try this with broccoli, bok choy, and mushrooms in place of the snow peas, carrots, and onions.

1. To make the Mongolian sauce, in a small bowl, whisk together the stock and cornstarch until dissolved. Whisk in the soy sauce, brown sugar, and sesame oil. Set aside.

2. To make the Mongolian beef, place the beef in a large bowl. Add the cornstarch and salt, place a lid on top of the bowl and shake until the beef is coated (or use a large, resealable plastic bag).

3. In a large sauté pan, skillet, or wok, heat the oil over medium heat. Add the beef and sauté for 3 to 4 minutes per side, until browned and crisp. Remove the beef from the pan and set aside.

4. Add the carrots, snow peas, and onion to the hot skillet and sauté for 3 to 4 minutes, until slightly soft. Put the beef back in the pan, as well as the ginger and garlic, stirring to sauté for 30 to 60 seconds, or until fragrant.

5. Add the sauce to the pan and bring to a simmer for 1 to 2 minutes, until thickened, stirring constantly.

6. Serve the Mongolian beef garnished with scallions (if using). Serve immediately.

7. The Mongolian beef can be prepped in advance and stored in airtight containers up to 3 days in the refrigerator. Reheat in the microwave 2 to 3 minutes or until heated through.

Per Serving: Calories: 302; Total fat: 15g; Saturated fat: 4g; Cholesterol: 56mg; Sodium: 607mg; Carbohydrates: 19g; Fiber: 2g; Sugar: 8g; Protein: 22g

Mediterranean Lamb Nachos

I used to make a time-intensive version of these lamb nachos at a restaurant I worked in several years ago. This is my quick weeknight version made with ground lamb and Middle Eastern spices, and it's totally delicious. I enjoy loading them up with cucumber, feta, olives, and a big dollop of Greek yogurt.

- 3 whole-grain pitas, cut into wedges
- 1 tablespoon avocado oil
  1 pound lean ground lamb
- 1-inch piece fresh ginger, peeled and minced
- 3 garlic cloves, peeled and minced
  1½ teaspoons ground coriander
  1 teaspoon ground cumin
  ½ teaspoon kosher or sea salt

½ teaspoon freshly ground black pepper
- ½ medium English cucumber, diced
- 1 pint cherry tomatoes, quartered
- ¼ cup sliced, pitted kalamata olives
  ¼ cup crumbled feta cheese
- ½ cup plain Greek yogurt

NUT-FREE

Serves: 6
Prep Time: 10 to 15 minutes
Cook Time: 10 to 15 minutes

Cooking tip
To make tzatziki sauce to serve on the nachos, combine 2 cups grated cucumber, 1½ cups plain Greek yogurt, 2 tablespoons extra-virgin olive oil, 2 tablespoons chopped fresh dill, zest and juice of ½ medium lemon, 1 minced garlic clove, and ½ teaspoon kosher or sea salt.

Variation tip
Try with ground turkey, chicken, or beef instead of lamb.

1. Preheat the oven to 400°F.
2. Place the pita wedges on a baking sheet and spritz with cooking spray. Bake for 8 to 10 minutes, or until lightly browned and crisp.
3. In a large sauté pan or skillet, heat the oil over medium heat. Add the lamb and sauté for 6 to 7 minutes, or until browned, breaking it up with a wooden spoon as it cooks. Drain the fat from the lamb and place it back in the hot skillet. Stir in the ginger, garlic, coriander, cumin, salt, and pepper and sauté for 30 to 60 seconds, or until fragrant.

4. Arrange the pita chips on plates and top with the lamb mixture, cucumbers, tomatoes, olives, feta, and dollops of Greek yogurt. Serve immediately.

5. The pita chips can be prepped in advance and stored in resealable bags for up to 3 days. The lamb mixture can be prepped in advance and stored in airtight containers for up to 4 days in the refrigerator. Reheat in the microwave for 2 to 3 minutes, or until heated through. Assemble the nachos just before serving.

Per Serving: Calories: 327; Total fat: 19g; Saturated fat: 5g; Cholesterol: 59mg; Sodium: 532mg; Carbohydrates: 24g; Fiber: 1g; Sugar: 3g; Protein: 18g

Mini Mixed-Berry Bread Puddings, Page 157

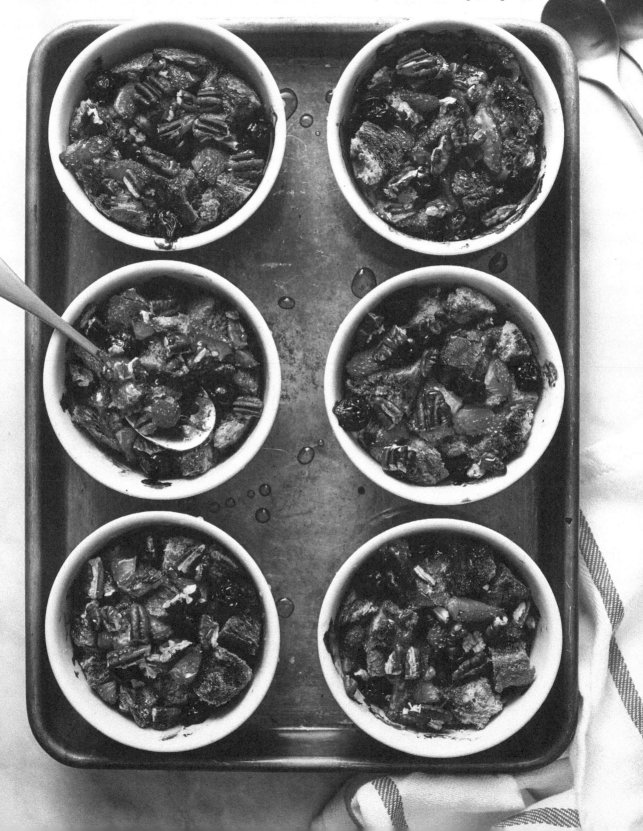

CHAPTER NINE

Healthy Desserts

Blueberry, Matcha, and Chia Seed Pudding

Matcha, which is finely ground green tea powder, is filled with flavonoids and antioxidants. In this application, it's mixed with chia seeds, milk, maple syrup, and vanilla to make a lightly sweetened pudding. Top it with blueberries and almonds for a delicious brain-supportive dessert.

1½ cups milk

½ cup canned full-fat coconut milk

▶ ½ cup chia seeds

¼ cup maple syrup or honey

1½ teaspoons pure vanilla extract

▶ 1 teaspoon matcha powder

¼ teaspoon kosher or sea salt

▶ 1 cup fresh blueberries

▶ ½ cup sliced almonds

GLUTEN-FREE VEGETARIAN

Serves: 6

Prep Time: 5 to 10 minutes, plus 4 hours refrigeration

Substitution tip
If you don't like coconut, simply omit it and add another ½ cup milk of choice.

Variation tip
Instead of matcha powder, use 2 teaspoons of chai tea from 2 tea bags.

1. In a medium bowl, whisk together the milk, coconut milk, chia seeds, maple syrup, vanilla extract, matcha, and salt until combined. Place a lid on the bowl and refrigerate at least 4 hours or until set.

2. Serve in dessert cups with blueberries and almonds on top.

3. Store chia pudding in airtight containers in the refrigerator up to 5 days.

Per Serving: Calories: 210; Total fat: 13g; Saturated fat: 4g; Cholesterol: 0mg; Sodium: 87mg; Carbohydrates: 20g; Fiber: 8g; Sugar: 7g; Protein: 5g

Pumpkin Coconut Mousse

Pumpkin mousse is the perfect fall treat, although I won't judge you if you enjoy it every season! With hints of cinnamon, nutmeg, and maple, this creamy, fluffy mousse will hit just the right note for your sweet tooth.

▶ ¼ cup cashews

▶ 1½ cups pumpkin purée

½ cup canned full-fat coconut milk

3 tablespoons maple syrup

1½ teaspoons ground cinnamon

1½ teaspoons pure vanilla extract

¼ teaspoon ground nutmeg

¼ teaspoon kosher or sea salt

GLUTEN-FREE
VEGAN

Serves: 4

Prep Time: 10 to 15 minutes, plus 1 hour chilling time

Cooking tip
Let the mixture run in the blender for a few extra minutes to make for extra fluffy mousse. Try it with honey instead of maple syrup.

Variation tip
Sauté 1 diced apple in 1 teaspoon of butter in a skillet on medium high until caramelized. Stir in ½ teaspoon ground cinnamon. Top mousse with sautéed cinnamon apples.

1. In a blender, combine the cashews and ½ cup water. Soak for 10 minutes, then drain the water.

2. To the blender, add the pumpkin purée, coconut milk, maple syrup, cinnamon, vanilla, nutmeg, and salt. Purée until very smooth, scraping the sides of the blender with a spatula as needed.

3. Pour into dessert glasses, cover, and refrigerate for at least 1 hour. Serve.

4. Store the pumpkin mousse in an airtight container in the refrigerator for up to 4 days.

Per Serving: Calories: 109; Total fat: 8g; Saturated fat: 5g; Cholesterol: 0mg; Sodium: 74mg; Carbohydrates: 8g; Fiber: 1g; Sugar: 2g; Protein: 2g

Peanut Butter No-Bake Cookies

No-bake cookies remind me of my childhood, but I can't say we were too concerned about the nutrition aspect of them. Sure, they were a treat and not something we ate regularly, but there's nothing wrong with upgrading dessert from a MIND diet perspective. These cookies have natural peanut butter, dark cocoa, and oats with a few suggestions for healthier mix-ins. YUM!

▶ ½ cup creamy peanut butter

¼ cup coconut oil

3 tablespoons granulated sugar

▶ 2 tablespoons dark cocoa powder

½ teaspoon pure vanilla extract

¼ teaspoon kosher or sea salt

▶ 1¾ cups quick-cooking oats

VEGAN

Makes 16 cookies

Prep Time: 10 to 15 minutes, plus 4 hours resting time

Substitution tip
Use gluten-free oats for gluten-free cookies.

Variation tip
Add ¼ cup mini dark chocolate chips, unsweetened shredded coconut, or raisins to the batter.

1. In a medium bowl, combine the peanut butter and coconut oil. Microwave for 1 minute, then stir until the coconut oil is fully melted. Stir in the sugar, cocoa powder, vanilla extract, and salt and mix well. Fold in the oats until combined.

2. Drop 1-tablespoon portions onto a sheet of parchment paper. Let sit 4 hours, or until hardened. Or, let sit in the refrigerator to allow the cookies to harden quickly.

3. Transfer to an airtight container, layering cookies with parchment paper, and store in the refrigerator up to 2 weeks.

Per Serving (1 cookie): Calories: 121; Total fat: 8g; Saturated fat: 4g; Cholesterol: 0mg; Sodium: 38mg; Carbohydrates: 11g; Fiber: 2g; Sugar: 4g; Protein: 3g

Peach and Oatmeal-Cookie Crisp

I call the topping on this crisp "oatmeal cookie" because the oats, butter, cinnamon, and brown sugar remind me of my favorite oatmeal cookies. While butter isn't a food we should eat daily, I absolutely love the taste of it in certain desserts, so with this recipe, I went for it. A little butter certainly won't hurt.

- ▸ 1 cup whole-wheat or oat flour
- ▸ 1 cup old-fashioned rolled oats
- 6 tablespoons cold butter, cubed
- ¼ cup dark brown sugar
- 1½ teaspoons ground cinnamon
- ½ teaspoon kosher or sea salt
- ▸ 6 medium peaches, cored and sliced (about 6 cups)
- ¼ cup granulated sugar
- 3 tablespoons cornstarch
- ▸ Zest and juice of ½ medium lemon (about 1 tablespoon each)
- 1 teaspoon pure vanilla extract

NUT-FREE
VEGETARIAN

Serves: 8
Prep Time: 10 to 15 minutes
Cook Time: 30 to 40 minutes

Substitution tip
For a vegan crisp, use coconut oil instead of butter.

Variation tip
Use 6 cups of berries instead of peaches, or a mix of 3 cups berries and 3 cups frozen, dark sweet cherries.

1. Preheat the oven to 375°F. Coat a 13-by-9-inch baking dish with cooking spray. Set aside.

2. In the bowl of a food processor, place the flour, oats, butter, brown sugar, cinnamon, and salt. Pulse the mixture while drizzling in 7 to 8 tablespoons of ice water, until the mixture comes together in large clumps.

3. In a large bowl, stir together the peaches, sugar, cornstarch, lemon zest and juice, and vanilla extract until combined. Transfer the peach mixture into the baking dish and spread in an even layer. Crumble the oat mixture on top of the peach mixture in an even layer.

4. Bake for 30 to 40 minutes, until the crust is lightly browned and the peaches are bubbly. Let sit for 5 to 10 minutes, then serve.

5. Store the crisp in an airtight container in the refrigerator for up to 5 days.

Per Serving: Calories: 262; Total fat: 10g; Saturated fat: 5g; Cholesterol: 23mg; Sodium: 73mg; Carbohydrates: 41g; Fiber: 4g; Sugar: 20g; Protein: 4g

Honey-Carrot Banana Bread

Who doesn't love banana bread? This version is sweetened with honey, uses several cups of shredded carrots, and is topped with a handful of nuts. Talk about a nutritional powerhouse of quick breads!

- 1¼ cups whole-wheat or oat flour
- ¼ cup almond flour or almond meal
- 2 tablespoons ground flaxseed
- 1 teaspoon ground cinnamon
- ¾ teaspoon baking powder
- ¾ teaspoon baking soda
- ½ teaspoon kosher or sea salt
- 2 medium ripe bananas, peeled (about 1 cup)
- ¾ cup honey or maple syrup
- ¼ cup avocado oil
- 2 large eggs
- 1½ teaspoons pure vanilla extract
- 2 cups peeled and shredded carrots
- ½ cup chopped walnuts or pecans

DAIRY-FREE
VEGETARIAN

Serves: 12

Prep Time: 10 to 15 minutes

Cook Time: 45 to 55 minutes

Substitution tip
Try shredded zucchini instead of carrots.

Cooking tip
Try whole-wheat pastry flour instead of regular whole-wheat flour for a more tender product.

1. Preheat the oven to 350°F. Coat a loaf pan with cooking spray. Set aside.

2. In a medium bowl, whisk together the flour, almond flour, flaxseed, cinnamon, baking powder, baking soda, and salt.

3. In another medium bowl, using a hand mixer on medium speed, whisk together the bananas, honey, and oil until fluffy. Whisk in the eggs, then the vanilla extract until thoroughly combined. On low speed, slowly add the dry ingredients to the banana mixture while whisking until just combined, scraping the sides of the bowl with a spatula as needed. Fold in the shredded carrots. Pour the mixture into the prepared loaf pan. Sprinkle the walnuts on top and lightly press into the batter.

4. Bake for 30 to 40 minutes, or until a toothpick inserted into the center comes out clean. Allow to cool, then slice and serve.

5. Store the banana bread in an airtight container at room temperature for up to 7 days.

Per Serving: Calories: 246; Total fat: 11g; Saturated fat: 1g; Cholesterol: 31mg; Sodium: 182mg; Carbohydrates: 35g; Fiber: 4g; Sugar: 22g; Protein: 5g

Dark Chocolate Mint Brownies

These brownies are rich, fudgy, and decadent—everything that makes brownies so "craveable" and delicious. A few drops of peppermint extract give them a hint of mint that makes the brownies extra special.

- 1 cup dark chocolate chips, divided
- ¼ cup coconut oil
- 2 large eggs, at room temperature
- ½ cup granulated sugar
- 1 teaspoon peppermint extract
- 1 cup almond flour or almond meal
- ¼ cup dark cocoa powder
- ¼ teaspoon kosher or sea salt

DAIRY-FREE
GLUTEN-FREE
VEGETARIAN

Makes 12 brownies
Prep Time: 10 to 15 minutes
Cook Time: 40 to 45 minutes

Cooking tip
Choose dark chocolate that is at least 80 percent cacao. Choose dark cocoa powder without added sugar.

Variation tip
Leave out the peppermint extract and swirl in a few tablespoons of warm peanut butter for peanut butter, dark chocolate brownies.

1. Preheat the oven to 375°F. Coat an 8-by-8-inch baking dish with cooking spray. Set aside.

2. In a medium bowl, combine ¾ cup of the chocolate chips and coconut oil. Microwave in 30-second increments, stirring in between, until the mixture is melted.

3. Place the eggs and sugar in a medium bowl and using a hand mixer on medium speed, beat for 5 to 7 minutes, or until fluffy and pale in color. Beat in the peppermint extract. Slowly pour the chocolate mixture into the sugar mixture until incorporated.

4. In a small bowl, whisk together the almond flour, cocoa powder, and salt until combined. Fold the dry ingredient mixture into the chocolate mixture until combined.

5. Transfer the batter to the prepared baking dish and sprinkle with the remaining ¼ cup chocolate chips. Bake for 40 to 45 minutes, or until set. Let cool, then slice and serve.

6. Store the brownies in an airtight container and store at room temperature up to 7 days.

Per Serving (1 brownie): Calories: 181; Total fat: 12g; Saturated fat: 5g; Cholesterol: 31mg; Sodium: 36mg; Carbohydrates: 18g; Fiber: 0g; Sugar: 15g; Protein: 4g

Mini Mixed-Berry Bread Puddings

Bread pudding reminds me of Christmas morning, but the addition of berries makes it seem like a summer dessert. So, essentially what I'm saying is it's a great all-around dessert that'll make you feel the warm and fuzzies. Plus, it's filled with brain-healthy nutrients from the berries, whole-grain bread, and nuts.

- ▶ 4 cups cubed whole-grain bread
- ▶ 2 cups fresh or frozen mixed berries
- ▶ 4 large eggs
- ½ cup milk
- 3 tablespoons granulated sugar
- 1½ teaspoons pure vanilla extract
- ½ teaspoon ground cinnamon
- ▶ ½ cup chopped walnuts or pecans
- 2 tablespoons maple syrup

VEGETARIAN

Serves: 8
Prep Time: 10 to 15 minutes
Cook Time: 20 to 25 minutes

Cooking tip
Use frozen berries so you can enjoy berry bread pudding year-round.

Variation tip
Use diced apples instead of berries.

1. Preheat the oven to 375°F. Coat 8 soufflé cups or ramekins with cooking spray. Set aside.
2. In a large bowl, mix together the bread cubes and berries.
3. In a separate medium bowl, whisk together the eggs, milk, sugar, vanilla extract, and cinnamon until well combined.
4. Distribute the bread-and-berry mixture into each soufflé cup. Divide the egg mixture between the cups. Top with walnuts. Bake for 20 to 25 minutes, or until the bread pudding is set.
5. Drizzle each with maple syrup and serve immediately.
6. Store bread puddings covered in the refrigerator for up to 7 days.

Per Serving: Calories: 243; Total fat: 8g; Saturated fat: 1g; Cholesterol: 93mg; Sodium: 182mg; Carbohydrates: 36g; Fiber: 3g; Sugar: 18g; Protein: 9g

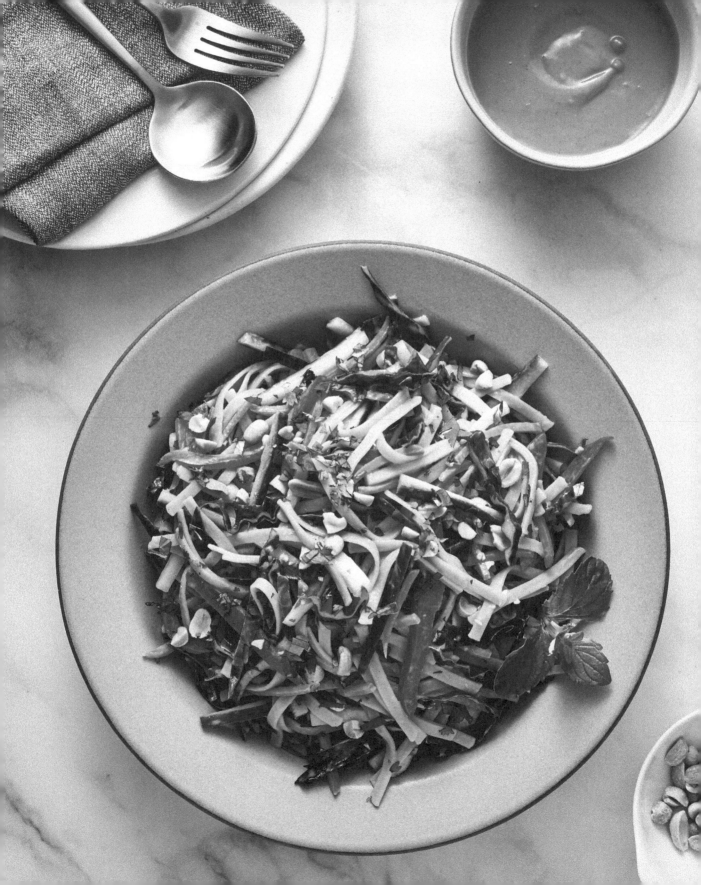

Measurement Conversions

	U.S. STANDARD	U.S. STANDARD (OUNCES)	METRIC (APPROXIMATE)
Volume Equivalents (Liquid)	2 tablespoons	1 fl. oz.	30 mL
	¼ cup	2 fl. oz.	60 mL
	½ cup	4 fl. oz.	120 mL
	1 cup	8 fl. oz.	240 mL
	1½ cups	12 fl. oz.	355 mL
	2 cups or 1 pint	16 fl. oz.	475 mL
	4 cups or 1 quart	32 fl. oz.	1 L
	1 gallon	128 fl. oz.	4 L
Volume Equivalents (Dry)	⅛ teaspoon	———	0.5 mL
	¼ teaspoon	———	1 mL
	½ teaspoon	———	2 mL
	¾ teaspoon	———	4 mL
	1 teaspoon	———	5 mL
	1 tablespoon	———	15 mL
	¼ cup	———	59 mL
	⅓ cup	———	79 mL
	½ cup	———	118 mL
	⅔ cup	———	156 mL
	¾ cup	———	177 mL
	1 cup	———	235 mL
	2 cups or 1 pint	———	475 mL
	3 cups	———	700 mL
	4 cups or 1 quart	———	1 L
	½ gallon	———	2 L
	1 gallon	———	4 L
Weight Equivalents	½ ounce	———	15 g
	1 ounce	———	30 g
	2 ounces	———	60 g
	4 ounces	———	115 g
	8 ounces	———	225 g
	12 ounces	———	340 g
	16 ounces or 1 pound	———	455 g

	FAHRENHEIT (F)	CELSIUS (C) (APPROXIMATE)
Oven Temperatures	250°F	120°C
	300°F	150°C
	325°F	180°C
	375°F	190°C
	400°F	200°C
	425°F	220°C
	450°F	230°C

Resources and References

RESOURCES

Andrews, Julie, MS, RDN, CD. *The MIND Diet Plan & Cookbook*. Emeryville, CA: Rockridge Press, 2019.

Morris, Martha Clare, Dr. *Diet for the MIND*. New York: Little, Brown and Company, 2017.

REFERENCES

Ahlskog, Eric, et al. "Physical exercise as a preventive or disease-modifying treatment of dementia and brain aging." *Mayo Clinic Proceedings*. 2011 Sep; 86(9): 876–884.

Ayaz M., et al. "Flavonoids as prospective neuroprotectants and their therapeutic propensity in aging associated neurological disorders." *Frontiers in Aging Neuroscience*. 2019 Jun; 11(155).

Bennett, David, et al. "Overview and findings from the Rush Memory and Aging Project." *Current Alzheimer's Research*. 2012 Jul 1; 9(6): 646–663.

Boccardi V., et al. "Beta-carotene, telomerase activity and Alzheimer's disease in old age subjects." *European Journal of Nutrition*. 2019 Jan.

Boyle, P.A., et al. "Effect of purpose in life on the relation between Alzheimer disease pathologic changes on cognitive function in advanced age." *Archives in General Psychiatry*. 2012 May; 69(5): 499–505.

Cahill, L. E., et al. "Fried-food consumption and risk of type 2 diabetes and coronary artery disease: A prospective study in 2 cohorts of US women and men." *American Journal of Clinical Nutrition*. 2014 Aug; 100(2): 667–675.

Cedars-Sinai. "Subjective Cognitive Impairment (SCI)." Accessed September 29, 2019. https://www.cedars-sinai.edu/Patients/Health-Conditions/Subjective-Cognitive-Impairment-SCI.aspx.

Cherian L., et al. "Mediterranean-DASH intervention for neurodegenerative delay (MIND) diet slows cognitive decline after stroke." *The Journal of Prevention of Alzheimer's Disease*. 2019 Jun; 6(4)267–273.

Cuomo, Alessandro, et al. "Depression and Vitamin D deficiency: causality, assessment, and clinical practice implications." *Neuropsychiatry.* 2017; 7(5): 606–614.

Devore, E. E, et al. "Dietary intakes of berries and flavonoids in relation to cognitive decline." *Annals of Neurology.* 2012 Jul; 72(1): 135–143.

Escher C, et al. "Stress and Alzheimer's disease." *Journal of Neural Transmission.* 2019 Feb 20; 126(9): 1155–1161.

Estruch R., et al. "Primary prevention of cardiovascular disease with a Mediterranean diet." *New England Journal of Medicine.* 2014 Feb; 370(9): 886.

Feart C., et al. "Associations of lower vitamin D concentrations with cognitive decline and long-term risk of dementia and Alzheimer's disease in older adults." *Alzheimer's and Dementia.* 2017; 13(11): 1207–1216.

Feart, C., et al. "Plasma carotenoids are inversely associated with dementia risk in an elderly French cohort." *The Journals of Gerontology.* 2016 May; 71(5): 683–688.

Fisher Center for Alzheimer's Research Foundation. "How a sense of purpose in life may help slow Alzheimer's." Accessed October 7, 2019. https://www.alzinfo.org/articles/sense-purpose-life-slow-alzheimers/.

Francis H., et al. "A brief diet intervention can reduce symptoms of depression in young adults—a randomized controlled trial." *Public Library of Science ONE.* 2019 Oct; 14(10).

Fultz N., et al. "Coupled electrophysiological, hemodynamic, and cerebrospinal fluid oscillations in human sleep." *Science.* 2019 Nov; 336(6465): 628–631.

Gomez-Pinilla F. "Brain foods: the effects of nutrients on brain function." *Nature Reviews Neuroscience.* 2008 Jul; 9(7): 568–578.

Gordon B., et al. "Association of efficacy of resistance exercise training with depressive symptoms." *Journal of the American Medical Association Psychiatry.* 2018 Jun; 75(6): 566–576.

Gottesman R., et al. "Associations between midlife vascular risk factors and 25-year incident dementia in the atherosclerosis risk in communities." *Journal of the American Medical Association Neurology.* 2017; 74(10): 1246–1254.

Hardman, R., et al. "Adherence to a Mediterranean-style diet and effects on cognition in adults: A qualitative evaluation and systematic review of longitudinal and prospective trials." *Frontiers in Nutrition.* 2016 July; 3: 22.

Harvard Health Publishing, Harvard Medical School. "Food and mood: Is there a connection?" Accessed October 6, 2019. https://www.health.harvard.edu/mind-and-mood/food-and-mood-is-there-a-connection.

Harvard Health Publishing, Harvard Medical School. "How memory and thinking ability change with age." Accessed October 5, 2019. https://www.health.harvard.edu/mind-and-mood/how-memory-and-thinking-ability-change-with-age.

Harvard Health Publishing, Harvard Medical School. "Understanding inflammation." Accessed October 9, 2019. https://www.health.harvard.edu/staying-healthy/understanding-inflammation.

Harvard T.H. Chan School of Public Health. "Three of the B Vitamins: Folate, Vitamin B6, and Vitamin B12." Accessed September 28, 2019. https://www.hsph.harvard.edu/nutritionsource/what-should-you-eat/vitamins/vitamin-b/.

Harvard T.H. Chan School of Public Health. "Vitamin E." Accessed October 9, 2019. https://www.hsph.harvard.edu/nutritionsource/vitamin-e/.

Healthline. "What causes dysbiosis and how is it treated?" Accessed October 11, 2019. https://www.healthline.com/health/digestive-health/dysbiosis.

Healthline. "What is choline? An essential nutrient with many benefits." Accessed October 12, 2019. https://www.healthline.com/nutrition/what-is-choline#sources.

Holzel B., et al. "Mindfulness practice leads to increases in regional brain gray matter density." *Psychiatry Research.* 2011 Jan; 191(1): 36–43.

Ju, Yo-El, et al. "Sleep and Alzheimer disease pathology: A bidirectional relationship." *Nature Reviews Neurology.* 2014; 10(2): 115–119.

Kowalski K., Mulak A. "Brain-gut-microbiota axis in Alzheimer's disease." *Journal of Neurogastroenterology and Motility*. 2019; 25(1): 48–60.

La Fata, Giorgio, et al. "Effects of vitamin E on cognitive performance during ageing and in Alzheimer's disease." *Nutrients*. 2014 Dec; 6(12): 5453–5472.

Larrieu, Thomas, et al. "Food for mood: relevance of nutritional omega-3 fatty acids for depression and anxiety." *Frontiers in Physiology*. 2018 Aug; 9(1047).

Lassale C., Batty D. G., et al. "Healthy dietary indices and risk of depressive outcomes: a systematic review and meta-analysis of observational studies." *Molecular Psychiatry*. 2019; 24(7): 965–986.

Lauritzen, Lotte, et al. "DHA effects in brain development and function." *Nutrients*. 2016 Jan; 8(1): 6.

Mayo Clinic. "Alzheimer's genes: are you at risk?" Accessed October 1, 2019. https://www.mayoclinic.org/diseases-conditions/alzheimers-disease/in-depth/alzheimers-genes/art-20046552.

Mayo Clinic. "Mild Cognitive Impairment (MCI)." Accessed September 30, 2019. https://www.mayoclinic.org/diseases-conditions/mild-cognitive-impairment/symptoms-causes/syc-20354578.

Mayo Clinic. "Mindfulness exercises." Accessed October 16, 2019. https://www.mayoclinic.org/healthy-lifestyle/consumer-health/in-depth/mindfulness-exercises/art-20046356.

Mayo Clinic. "Red wine and resveratrol: Good for your heart?" Accessed October 1, 2019. https://www.mayoclinic.org/diseases-conditions/heart-disease/in-depth/red-wine/art-20048281.

Mayo Clinic. "Water: Essential to your body." Accessed October 1, 2019. https://mayoclinichealthsystem.org/hometown-health/speaking-of-health/water-essential-to-your-body.

McEvoy, C. T., et al. "Neuroprotective diets are associated with better cognitive function: The health and retirement study." *Journal of the American Geriatrics Society*. 2017 Aug; 65(8): 1857–1862.

McGarel C., et al. "Emerging roles for folate and related B-vitamins in brain health across the lifecycle." *Proceedings of the Nutrition Society.* 2015 Feb; 74(1): 46–55.

Medline Plus. "Aging changes in sleep." Accessed October 12, 2019. https://medlineplus.gov/ency/article/004018.htm.

Miller, M. G., et al. "Dietary blueberry improves cognition among older adults in a randomized, double-blind, placebo-controlled trial." *European Journal of Nutrition.* 2018 Apr; 57(3): 1169–1180.

Mock, J. Thomas, et al. "The influence of vitamins E and C and exercise on brain aging." *Experimental Gerontology.* 2017 Aug; 94: 69–72.

Morris, M. C. "The role of nutrition in Alzheimer's disease: epidemiological evidence." *European Journal of Neurology.* 2009 Sep; 16(Suppl 1): 1–7.

Morris, M. C., et al. "Associations of vegetable and fruit consumption with age-related cognitive change." *Neurology.* 2006 Oct 24; 67(8): 1370–1376.

Morris, M. C., et al. "Dietary fats and the risk of incident Alzheimer's disease." *Archives of Neurology.* 2003 Aug; 60(8): 1072.

Morris, M. C., et al. "Vitamin E and cognitive decline in older persons." *Archives of Neurology.* 2002 Jul; 59(7): 1125–1132.

Morris, Martha Clare, et al. "Consumption of fish and n-3 fatty acids and risk of incident Alzheimer's disease." *Archives of Neurology.* 2003; 60(7): 940–946.

Morris, Martha Clare, et al. "MIND diet associated with reduced incidence of Alzheimer's disease." *Alzheimer's & Dementia.* 2015 Sep; 11(9): 1007–1014.

Morris, Martha Clare, et al. "MIND diet slows cognitive decline with aging." *Alzheimer's & Dementia.* 2016 Sep; 11(9): 1015–1022.

Morris, Martha Clare, Dr. *Diet for the MIND.* New York: Little, Brown and Company, 2017.

Mullan, K., et al. "Serum concentrations of vitamin E and carotenoids are altered in Alzheimer's disease: A case-control study." *Alzheimer's & Dementia.* 2017 Jul 19; 3(3): 432–439.

Naqvi, Asghar, et al. "Monounsaturated, trans, and saturated fatty acids and cognitive decline in women." *Journal of the American Geriatrics Society*. 2011 May; 59(5): 837–843.

National Institute on Aging. "A good night's sleep." Accessed October 5, 2019. https://www.nia.nih.gov/health/good-nights-sleep.

National Institute on Aging. "Alzheimer's disease genetics fact sheet." Accessed on September 27, 2019. https://www.nia.nih.gov/health/alzheimers-disease-genetics-fact-sheet.

National Institute on Aging. "How the aging brain affects thinking." Accessed October 1, 2019. https://www.nia.nih.gov/health/how-aging-brain-affects-thinking.

National Institute on Aging. "Preventing Alzheimer's disease: What do we know?" Accessed on October 3, 2019. https://www.nia.nih.gov/health/preventing-alzheimers-disease-what-do-we-know.

National Institute on Aging. "What is Alzheimer's disease?" Accessed September 30, 2019. https://www.nia.nih.gov/health/what-alzheimers-disease.

National Institute on Aging. "What is Dementia? Symptoms, types, and diagnosis." Accessed September 29, 2019. https://www.nia.nih.gov/health/what-dementia-symptoms-types-and-diagnosis.

National Institutes of Health. "Risk factors for heart disease linked to dementia." Accessed September 28, 2019. https://www.nih.gov/news-events/nih-research-matters/risk-factors-heart-disease-linked-dementia.

National Institutes of Health. "Vitamin D." Accessed October 10, 2019. https://ods.od.nih.gov/factsheets/VitaminD-HealthProfessional/.

Oregon State University. "Flavonoids." Accessed October 3, 2019. https://lpi.oregonstate.edu/mic/dietary-factors/phytochemicals/flavonoids.

Owaga E., et al. "Nutritional management of mental disorders: Potential role of dietary flavonoids and vitamin E." *Food and Public Health*. 2014; 4(3): 104–109.

Poly C, Massaro J. M., et al. "The relation of dietary choline to cognitive performance and white-matter hyperintensity in the Framingham Offspring Cohort." *American Journal of Clinical Nutrition*. 2011 Dec; 94(6): 1584–1591.

Romagnolo, Donato. "Mediterranean diet and prevention of chronic diseases." *Nutrition Today*. 2017 Sep; 52(5): 208–22.

Shukitt-Hale B., et al. "Blueberries improve neuroinflammation and cognition differentially depending on individual cognitive baseline status." *The Journals of Gerontology*. 2019 Jul; 74(7): 977–983.

Stringham J., et al. "Lutein across the lifespan: from childhood cognitive performance to the aging eye and brain." *Current Developments in Nutrition*. 2019 Jul; 3(7).

Travica, N., et al. "Plasma vitamin C concentrations and cognitive function: a cross-sectional study." *Frontiers in Aging Neuroscience*. 2019 Apr; 11:72.

Tyndall A., et al. "Protective effects of exercise on cognition and brain health in older adults." *Exercise and Sport Sciences Review*. 2018 Oct; 46(4): 215–223.

U.S. News & World Report. "What is DASH Diet?" Accessed October 2, 2019. https://health.usnews.com/best-diet/dash-diet.

University of Michigan Health. "How diet influences mood and mental health." Accessed October 6, 2019. https://healthblog.uofmhealth.org/lifestyle/how-diet -influences-mood-and-mental-health.

USDA. "Dietary guidelines for Americans 2015 2020." September 26, 2019. https://www.choosemyplate.gov/dietary-guidelines.

Vasanthi, Hannah, et al. "Health benefits of wine and alcohol from neuroprotection to heart health." *Frontiers in Bioscience*. 2012 Jan; 4: 1505–1512.

Weiser, Michael, et al. "Docosahexaenoic acid and cognition throughout the lifespan." *Nutrients*. 2016 Feb; 8(2): 99.

Wengreen H., et al. "Prospective study of Dietary Approaches to Stop Hypertension- and Mediterranean-style dietary patterns and age-related cognitive change: The Cache County Study on memory, health and aging." *American Journal of Clinical Nutrition*. 2013 Nov; 98(5): 1263–71.

Williams K., et al. "Exploring interventions to reduce cognitive decline in aging." *Journal of Psychosocial Nursing and Mental Health Services*. 2011 May; 48(5): 42–51.

Wilson, R. S., et al. "Proneness to psychological distress is associated with risk of Alzheimer's disease." *Neurology*. 2003 Dec; 61(11): 1479–85.

Yuan, Changzheng, et al. "Long-term intake of vegetables and fruits and subjective cognitive function in US men." *Neurology*. 2019 Jan; 92(1): 63–75.

Zuniga K., et al. "Relationship between dietary lutein and cognition in an older adult population." *Current Developments in Nutrition*. 2019 Jun; 3(1).

INDEX

Page locators, bold italic (*02*), indicate photograph.

ACKNOWLEDGMENTS

To Ben, my feisty, adventurous, and witty husband, who is the most supportive person in my life. You've always encouraged me and indulged in my wild and crazy dreams, and I'll always be grateful for that. XO.

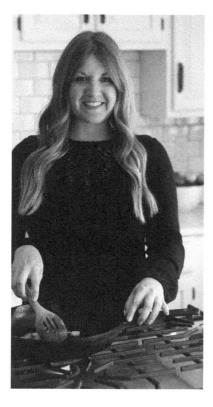

ABOUT THE AUTHOR

Julie Andrews, MS, RDN, CD, is a registered dietitian nutritionist and trained chef with a master's degree in human nutrition. She is a food and nutrition consultant, recipe developer, food photographer, media chef, and food writer. She authored *The MIND Diet Plan & Cookbook* and *The Simple Soups Cookbook*, and co-authored *The 28-Day DASH Diet Weight-Loss Program*. She shares simple, wholesome, and delicious recipes on her blog, TheGourmetRD.com.